DSM-5-TR®
POCKET GUIDE
FOR
CHILD AND ADOLESCENT MENTAL HEALTH

DSM-5-TR®
POCKET GUIDE
FOR
CHILD AND ADOLESCENT MENTAL HEALTH

by

Robert J. Hilt, M.D.

*Professor of Psychiatry, University of Washington,
and Director of Partnership Access Line, Seattle
Children's, Seattle, Washington*

Abraham M. Nussbaum, M.D.

*Professor of Psychiatry and Assistant Dean of
Graduate Medical Education, University of Colorado
School of Medicine, and Chief Education Officer,
Denver Health, Aurora, Colorado*

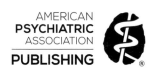

AMERICAN
PSYCHIATRIC
ASSOCIATION
PUBLISHING

Note: The authors have worked to ensure that all information in this book is accurate at the time of publication and consistent with general psychiatric and medical standards, and that information concerning drug dosages, schedules, and routes of administration is accurate at the time of publication and consistent with standards set by the U.S. Food and Drug Administration and the general medical community. As medical research and practice continue to advance, however, therapeutic standards may change. Moreover, specific situations may require a specific therapeutic response not included in this book. For these reasons and because human and mechanical errors sometimes occur, we recommend that readers follow the advice of physicians directly involved in their care or the care of a member of their family.

Books published by American Psychiatric Association Publishing represent the findings, conclusions, and views of the individual authors and do not necessarily represent the policies and opinions of American Psychiatric Association Publishing or the American Psychiatric Association.

If you wish to buy 50 or more copies of the same title, please go to www.appi.org/specialdiscounts for more information.

Copyright © 2025 American Psychiatric Association Publishing

ALL RIGHTS RESERVED

First Edition

Manufactured in the United States of America on acid-free paper
28   27   26   25   24   5   4   3   2   1

American Psychiatric Association Publishing
800 Maine Avenue SW, Suite 900
Washington, DC 20024–2812
www.appi.org

Library of Congress Cataloging-in-Publication Data
Names: Hilt, Robert J., 1969– author. | Nussbaum, Abraham M., 1975– author. | American Psychiatric Association, issuing body.
Title: DSM-5-TR pocket guide to child and adolescent mental health / by Robert J. Hilt, Abraham M. Nussbaum.
Other titles: Pocket guide for child and adolescent mental health
Description: First edition. | Washington, D.C. : American Psychiatric Association Publishing, [2025] | Includes bibliographical references and index.
Identifiers: LCCN 2024013483 (print) | LCCN 2024013484 (ebook) | ISBN 9781615375462 (paperback) | ISBN 9781615375479 (ebook)
Subjects: MESH: Diagnostic and statistical manual of mental disorders (Fifth edition, text revision) | Mental Disorders—diagnosis | Child | Mental Disorders—therapy | Adolescent | Interview, Psychological—methods | Handbook
Classification: LCC RJ503 (print) | LCC RJ503 (ebook) | NLM WS 39 | DDC 616.8900835—dc23/eng/20240416
LC record available at https://lccn.loc.gov/2024013483
LC ebook record available at https://lccn.loc.gov/2024013484

British Library Cataloguing in Publication Data
A CIP record is available from the British Library.

Contents

PART I
MEETING, DIAGNOSING, AND TREATING CHILDREN AND ADOLESCENTS

PART II
ENGAGING CHILDREN AND ADOLESCENTS WITH DSM-5-TR

PART III
ADDITIONAL TOOLS AND
CLINICAL GUIDANCE

Preface

You help children and adolescents when you seek understanding of their distress with the *Diagnostic and Statistical Manual of Mental Disorders*, Fifth Edition, Text Revision (DSM-5-TR; American Psychiatric Association 2022). When you comprehend a child or adolescent's distress, you advance the mental health care they receive, directing them, variously, to academic supports, community engagement, psychotherapy, medications, and more. Yet offering such direction can feel impossible when you meet a child or adolescent because their health is so bound up with the communities and families in which they are situated.

When you prudently use DSM-5-TR, you obtain an evidence-based and consensus-driven account of the mental distress experienced by the child or adolescent before you. You determine their age and their developmental age. You learn their temperament and the temperament of their parents. You explore the health of their family and community. But DSM-5-TR is a manual for diagnosing mental illness in a particular person, so using it with children and adolescents, whose health is inevitably bound up in culture, ethnicity, faith, family history, gender, medical history, sexual orientation, race, and temperament, requires interpretation. We offer this pocket guide as a pragmatic translation of DSM-5-TR for effective treatment.

We interview patients with students, trainees, and fellow practitioners every day, so we wrote this book for interviewers at all levels of experience. The first part of the book introduces the diagnostic interview, its goals, and how to structure an interview on the basis of how much time you have with a person. The second part operationalizes the DSM-5-TR diagnostic criteria for clinical practice. The third part includes additional information, tables, and tools. Taken as a whole, this book helps you accurately diagnose mental disorders in a child or an adolescent while establishing a therapeutic alliance, which remains the goal of any psychiatric encounter.

Before we begin, a few words about language. When possible, we use gender-neutral terms for the person and the interviewer, but when doing so is grammatically awkward, we use the singular *they*.

Wherever possible, we emphasize a child or adolescent's agency, their ability to act in the world. To signal this emphasis, we use the word *person* to describe the object of mental health evaluation. We acknowledge that a robust debate exists around whether the object of medical care is best construed as an ill patient under the care of a health professional or as an autonomous consumer of that professional's services (Emanuel and Emanuel 1992). Personhood precedes illness, or any other identity, so we prefer *person*. However, when we write about a person who has entered psychiatric treatment, we use the term *patient*. By using *patient*, we are not endorsing medical paternalism but acknowledging the vulnerability of the person in treatment and the responsibilities assumed by professionals when they care for patients (Radden and Sadler 2010). We use *patient* to emphasize that the particular and protected relationships that develop in clinical encounters are better described as therapeutic relationships between patients and clinicians than as therapeutic contracts between consumers and providers.

Because children and adolescents often depend on a variety of adults—parents, extended family members, adult friends, teachers, faith leaders, coaches, and more—we use the term *caregiver* to describe an adult who cares for a child or an adolescent outside of medical relationships.

Finally, we are both physicians, but children and adolescents receive care within medical relationships from persons trained in a variety of helping professions. To acknowledge this variety, we use the term *clinician* to describe a medical professional who cares for children and adolescents while constantly practicing and refining their craft.

Acknowledgments

We thank the teachers and students with whom we learned (and still learn) how to care for children and adolescents in mental distress, our respective academic and clinical homes for encouraging this work, and our own families for tolerating our efforts.

The authors have no competing interests or conflicts to declare.

PART I

Meeting, Diagnosing, and Treating Children and Adolescents

Chapter 1

Starting Out With a Therapeutic Alliance

Right as your overbooked morning session is ending, you are asked to assess the mental health of Sophie, a distressed 14-year-old girl you have never met. You gather yourself, enter her examination room, and find a poorly groomed girl with her arms crossed over her chest, staring up at the ceiling rather than looking at you. She says to no one in particular, "There is nothing wrong, and I don't need to be here." Her mother speaks for her, describing school struggles, arguments at home, losing friends, and saying "strange" things that include threats to hurt herself and talking to herself when she is alone. She says Sophie has a history of maltreatment by her mother's previous boyfriend, and in subsequent years she has had "mood swings." As her mother speaks, Sophie picks at the scabs overlaying the linear lacerations on her left forearm.

That sinking feeling you just experienced—the time-stressed challenge of how to skillfully assess mental health concerns in a pediatric population—is something we have experienced too. We wrote this book to be the guide you take with you as you journey with patients like Sophie.

What Is in This Book?

Like *The Pocket Guide to the DSM-5-TR® Diagnostic Exam* (Nussbaum 2022), this book emphasizes a person-centered approach to diagnosis through practical tools and concise interview guides. What sets this book apart is that all its tools are designed specifically for children and their caregivers, and it helps you navigate from diagnosis to treatment in any setting. After all, young people are more likely than adults to receive an initial mental health diagnosis and treatment in non–behavioral health settings, so we pay particular attention to what you can perform practically in any setting during clinical encounters such as the following:

- Assessing a child or adolescent in crisis (Chapter 3)
- Diagnostically investigating common complaints (Chapter 4)
- Performing either brief 15-minute (Chapter 5) or longer 30-minute (Chapter 6) versions of a diagnostic interview
- Rating mental health symptoms and treatment responses (Chapters 11 and 12)
- Recognizing developmental milestones (Chapter 13)
- Initiating initial psychosocial (Chapter 15), psychotherapeutic (Chapter 16), and psychopharmacological (Chapter 17) intervention

When you read the book in its entirety, you will develop multiple approaches to caring for young people. When you read a specific section, it will be your in-the-moment guide, offering the right interview questions to investigate a specific DSM-5-TR (American Psychiatric Association 2022) diagnosis and directing you to the most evidence-based initial treatments. To help you along the way, the book includes the following:

- A focus on the diagnoses experienced by children and adolescents
- The exclusion of diagnoses not commonly made in childhood or adolescence
- Brief chapters and practical tables
- Assessment tools specifically for children and adolescents
- ICD-10 codes for diagnoses

We developed each clinical tool out of our own experiences. We remember struggling through encounters with children and adolescents, wondering how to organize the disparate symptoms and concerns we heard. We benefited from other interview guides (e.g., Cepeda and Gotanco 2017; Youngstrom et al. 2022) and eventually developed a variety of ways to organize a diagnostic and treatment encounter even in time-constrained circumstances.

As coauthors, we have served in different postresidency clinical roles that include being a rural pediatrician, a pediatric hospitalist, a pediatric emergency physician, a child psychiatrist, a child psychiatric consultant to both tertiary care and rural pediatricians, and an adult inpatient psychiatrist. We provided psychotherapy and medication treatments for young people and adapted what we do for the shifting needs and structures of various care settings. In the course of this work, we have been humbled by the challenges young people face and the challenges they present to the person who dares to offer mental health assistance. After all, few children and adolescents arrive on our doorsteps with neatly described symptoms that map perfectly onto the symptom list of a single DSM-5-TR disorder. We have both made mistakes in our diagnostic processes with young people and have grown from those experiences.

The resulting book is an experience-based guide to child mental health diagnosis and treatment intended to provide a variety of practical approaches, tips, and skills to supplement the diagnostic content of DSM-5-TR. We cannot offer any rigid rules to follow when diagnosing or treating mental health disorders in young people because good care for young people cannot be reduced to a checklist. Whatever your specialty, your practice setting, and your experience level, we assist you as you journey with children and adolescents pursuing mental health.

Therapeutic Alliance: The Place to Start

When meeting a clinician for the first time, young people are often reluctant participants. Some may have developmentally limited communication skills. Many have been presented for care that they did not seek on their own. All will require you to gather information from multiple informants and construct an age- and developmentally adjusted differential diagnosis.

Corresponding to the patient's reluctance is often a clinician's anxiety about how they will prudently account for the person before them, especially when working in settings with time-limited evaluations. A clinician's sense of a ticking clock increases the challenges of efficiently arriving at a diagnosis and treatment plan for a young person.

For the patient and clinician alike, the first step in successful diagnosis and treatment is to support the collaborative treatment relationship, the *therapeutic alliance*, with the patient and their caregivers. Consider the 14-year-old girl in the vignette at the beginning of this chapter, Sophie. Sophie communicates that she disagrees with her mother's assessment of the situation and is disinterested in your services. If you were to just open DSM-5-TR and start reading out diagnostic criteria questions to Sophie, it would likely only increase her resistance.

If we were in the examination room with you, we would hear out the concerns of Sophie's mother, which solidifies the parental therapeutic alliance; we would thank her for the guidance; and we would tell her that after hearing the concerns of caregivers, we speak with all our adolescent patients alone. We would describe the rules for that discussion—namely, that the conversation is confidential except for safety concerns—and then invite Sophie to sit alone with us. We do this because you develop a better alliance; you obtain more honest answers when you interview adolescents without a parent or caregiver present (Ford et al. 1997; Gold and Seningen 2009). However, this guidance must be adapted to each situation; a separation should not be forced on adolescents who do not want their caregivers to leave the room. Younger children, or those adolescents who appear to be developmentally immature, are usually interviewed more successfully with caregivers present and reassuring them.

All young people will have a better therapeutic alliance if they feel noticed, heard, and appreciated, through *empathic engagement*. Even clinicians in a time-pressured situation should be reassured that holding back a recitation of targeted diagnostic questions to really notice the patient and build a little engagement does not take long. In our experience, creating an engaged therapeutic alliance up front with a reluctant interviewee saves time overall through enhanced cooperation with the diagnostic process.

Starting with a genuine reflecting statement that follows someone's lead can initiate engagement with an adolescent, such as saying to Sophie, *"You said that you feel fine and that there is nothing wrong. I would like to hear more about what is going well for you right now...."* You could also start the conversation by asking about something that is important to the patient but relatively situation-neutral, such as, *"Your mom said that you go to _____ school; what is that school like?"* School, friends, family, and favorite activities can all be appropriate and relatively low-stress conversation starters. If they are not, try asking about a favorite book, activity, or sports team. Sometimes we ask about something a patient brings into the room, such as stickers on a water bottle or the logo on a T-shirt. Pursue whichever subject induces the patient to speak freely with an inviting emotional tone.

When young persons seem reluctant to even start talking, you may find that the conversation flows better after you describe something you saw. This shows that you have been paying attention to them. For instance, *"It looked as if it was really hard to just sit there and do nothing while your mom was talking. Am I right about that?"* If there is a chance to comment on something you saw that relates to the diagnostic theme, you could also take that opportunity, saying, for example, *"I saw you shake your head when your mom described what happened yesterday. Did she say something that wasn't true for you?"*

With a very young child, a conversation starter could be a simple observation, such as a comment about what they are wearing or brought with them, such as, *"I see you have flowers on your shoes; did you pick those out yourself?"* You can also comment on something the young person is currently doing, such as how they are playing with a toy or drawing a picture, to start a conversation.

A subtler strategy to build the treatment alliance with a young person is to shape how you speak in a way that shows that you will be a responsive, problem-solving partner rather than an authority who will judge them. Metaphorically speaking, this is about getting you and your young patient to sit side by side to talk through a problem together. That way, the young person can talk about a problem that does not involve who they are as a person. For instance, Sophie may feel less defensive if you conversationally refer to her "mood" having led her to cut herself rather than stating "you cut yourself."

A bit of humor can sometimes help get young people talking. If humor does not come easily to you, be aware that showing some humility about yourself can be disarming and get your patient to chuckle a little. Both of us have children of our own who daily remind us that we have not been "cool" for a long time (if we ever were), and we find that openly acknowledging our status as uncool adults can humanize us and put a young person at ease. For instance, *"What is that band's name on your shirt? I have not heard about them before, but that probably means they are cool because I am a bit of a square."* As you meet a patient, stick to self-deprecating humor: make yourself, not your new patient, the punchline.

Building a therapeutic alliance with a young person should lead to learning a young patient's own true chief complaint. For Sophie, it could be "My mom is driving me crazy,"

"My boyfriend is abusive," "I hear voices," or any of several complaints. This creates a context from which your subsequent and more detailed diagnostic inquiries will logically follow. Following conversational opportunities can go like this: "*So, during those times when your mom is driving you crazy, do you ever have thoughts about hurting yourself?*" Child and parent chief complaints do not have to align; we have performed many successful treatments from start to finish with young people whose chief complaints never fully aligned with what their parents thought the problem was.

Once you have the young person engaged and talking with you, the diagnostic and treatment process as described throughout the rest of this book will follow more easily. It is our experience that once a reasonable therapeutic alliance is initiated, your patient will answer your questions about what they see as the challenges in their life more honestly. You can enter the territory of their mental life together.

In summary, we suggest the following techniques for initiating a therapeutic alliance with a child and setting up a useful diagnostic interview:

- Prepare briefly before entering the room by reviewing available records to focus on the "why now," the reason for today's encounter.
- When developmentally appropriate, offer to talk with the patient without a caregiver present.
- Start the conversation with an observation or a subject important to the patient.
- Briefly convey that you have noticed, heard, and appreciated the patient's perspective.
- Show that you are the child's treatment partner rather than an adult-engaged adjudicator.
- Use self-deprecating humor to break the ice, such as confessing your "uncoolness."
- Ask about the patient's main concerns or frustrations.
- Try shaping your initial diagnostic questions to reference the child's own chief complaint.

Chapter 2

Meeting a Young Person Experiencing Mental Distress

Across the globe, children infrequently receive timely care for mental and behavioral health problems. This problem has long been recognized. Decades ago, researchers in the United States found that the average time from the start of mental health symptoms until a young person entered mental health treatment was 8–10 years (Kessler et al. 2005). In many systems of care, only about one in five children with a diagnosable mental health disorder received treatment during childhood (U.S. Public Health Service 1999). Among those children identified in primary care settings as needing a behavioral health intervention, a little more than half of those referred to a specialist will attend even a single treatment appointment (Rushton et al. 2002). In a more recent survey of children with mental health care needs across Europe, it was found that 32% in high-resourced countries and 19% in low-resourced countries had received any mental health treatment over the preceding 12 months (Kovess-Masfety et al. 2017).

The reasons for underuse of specific mental health treatments during childhood are numerous. Barriers include stigma, poor problem recognition, limited family or clinician understanding of treatments, insurance coverage barriers, complicated referral processes, and limited availability of mental health specialists.

There are far more community issues than any individual clinician can address. Thankfully, opportunities are now increasing for clinicians to participate in meaningful improvements in community behavioral health systems. Through payer supports and system redesigns, primary care practices or school health centers may be able to develop collaborative or integrated care partnerships with mental health specialists. Doing so brings specialist support directly into sites where young people are already receiving medical services. Research has determined that such arrangements can be clinically more effective and even save money for the overall care system, a fact that has captured the attention of health systems and payers.

Regardless of the specific system of care available in your community, we emphasize certain general clinical steps that appear along the path of addressing child behavioral health problems in community settings. If you are a primary care clinician or a health system representative working to improve community behavioral health, identifying opportunities to improve any of the following areas is likely to improve the health of children:

- Recognition of mental distress
- Screening for mental distress
- Diagnosis of a particular mental disorder
- Education about mental health treatment
- Teaching self-help strategies to patients and caregivers
- Initiation of counseling and therapy
- Appropriate prescription of medications

Recognition of Mental Distress

Before a child can receive services, they first must be *recognized* as needing some form of assistance. Caregivers differ greatly in their view of what requires professional help. The same set of disruptive behaviors may lead one caregiver to write it off as "Oh, he's just being a kid" but another caregiver to demand to see a professional. Families may actively resist acknowledging or may simply fail to recognize when the child has a problem that treatment could help. Therefore, a key initial step in the process is for family members, friends, school representatives, and primary care clinicians to help parents recognize what can and cannot be helped through mental health treatment and overcome barriers related to stigma when necessary. Education about general signs of trouble to watch for—such as worsening school performance or a loss of the ability to have fun—can aid with problem recognition.

Screening for Mental Distress

Proactively looking for mental health problems through direct questioning or evaluating symptoms with a behavioral health rating scale is worthwhile if clinicians are available to interpret that information and recommend appropriate actions. Rating scales are useful because they are easy to administer and enable the clinician to identify unrecognized problems, to obtain clinical data from multiple informants, and to receive assessments of symptom severity to follow.

Rating scales are imperfect; they should never be the sole basis for making a diagnosis because questions might be misinterpreted, be answered untruthfully, or simply be the wrong questions to ask. For instance, an adolescent with recent-onset inattention problems may have a depressive disorder or an anxiety disorder that is missed or misdiagnosed if the only diagnostic assessment used is an attention-deficit/hyperactivity disorder (ADHD) symptom rating scale. An adolescent who denies having depressive symptoms on a rating scale but is engaging in recurrent self-harm and otherwise presents with signs and symptoms of depressive disorder should still receive specialized care. The most valuable steps in the screening process are selecting the correct rating scales, interpreting the results in the context of a person's overall personal situation, and taking helpful action for any positive screening results.

Diagnosis of a Particular Mental Disorder

Making a mental health diagnosis and developing a treatment plan can be challenging for a mental health care clinician who has an hour to complete an assessment. For those who are less experienced or have only 15 minutes to assess a person, the task can be overwhelming. Within a very short time frame, all that we would reasonably ask of a clinician is to engage the child in further care by identifying the child's leading problem and its probable rather than definitive origin.

A well-supported DSM-5-TR (American Psychiatric Association 2022) diagnosis requires three things: 1) that a child's clinical presentation fulfills the specific symptom-based diagnostic criteria, 2) that those symptoms are not caused by other diagnoses or stressors, and 3) that those symptoms are impairing the child's functioning. Because it is challenging to make an accurate diagnosis, we recommend breaking the process into several steps. We recommend that in an initial brief assessment with incomplete information clinicians consider using less specific diagnoses, such as unspecified disruptive, impulse-control, and conduct disorders or unspecified depressive disorder. The diagnosis then can be clarified over time through the gathering of more information at subsequent appointments. This multistep approach allows the time needed to gather collateral information for subsequent review, such as data from ADHD rating scales completed by both teachers and family members.

When a clinician identifies multiple problems in an initial brief appointment, working with a young person and their caregivers to jointly identify the leading problem allows for a more practical use of time. For instance, if a child is having screaming tantrums, is hitting other children, is sleeping poorly, and sometimes appears anxious, the identified leading problem may be the unsafe externalizing behaviors. In that case, the child's sleep problems and intermittent anxiety might be set aside to explore further at a future appointment.

Education About Mental Health Treatment

Educating children and families about their diagnosed mental health disorders is intrinsically valuable. Besides fulfilling an inherent desire to better understand problems, providing psychoeducation increases the child's and caregiver's ability to achieve health. Resistance to bringing a child to see a mental health clinician or to trying out an appropriate psychiatric medication is common. So even if you make the best diagnosis possible, it does little good unless you connect the diagnosis to treatment. We keep the timeless advice of the physician Henry Cohen (1943) in mind: "All diagnoses are provisional formulae designed for action" (p. 24).

Seeking the right action educates patients and caregivers about the value of receiving mental health services. This helps a patient and their caregivers visualize the process of treatment, what is known about the anticipated response to treatment, and what is likely to happen without treatment. For instance, we might help a caregiver who is reluctant to see a mental health specialist understand that it takes an episode of untreated major depression an average of about 8 months to resolve on its own, which, if that happens, is a great deal of life and typical development for a child to miss out on (Birmaher et al. 2007). For a family who, because of the child's dysfunction, has lost some of their empathy for their child (which can happen with externalizing problems such as oppositional defiant disorder), providing blame-free psychoeducation about the condition and the likelihood of response to treatment can also reestablish caregiver empathy and support.

Teaching Self-Care Strategies to Patients and Caregivers

If a primary care clinician defers to a mental health clinician to initiate all forms of intervention, care is delayed for a young person. Delays can occur from stigma-related resistance, challenges in negotiating insurance restrictions, and waiting for a clinician to become available. We prefer that some form of treatment plan initiation occur right away once a disorder is identified, through the kind of steps that would be appropriate for a primary care clinician to recommend.

What would be appropriate treatment to recommend without a mental health clinician? The first step in treatment plan initiation could be coaching the child and family on self-help measures they can implement now. For example, the clinician could address a young person's poor sleep habits, which accompany many different mental and behavioral health problems. Coaching about sleep hygiene, such as restricting access to text messaging after a certain time of night, can reduce daytime irritability and improve mood, as we discuss in Chapter 15, "Initiating Psychosocial Interventions."

We also recommend a few situation-specific self-help readings or videos, which are sometimes called *bibliotherapy*. Behavior management training for disruptive behavior is a prime example because we know that a motivated parent can make significant changes in a child's discipline plan and environment from such interactions, without a therapist's involvement (Lavigne et al. 2008). Many high-quality books, websites, and videos are available for motivated parents to try implement evidence-based disruptive behavior management or skills informed by cognitive-behavioral therapy. However, even when parents use high-quality self-care tools, this is less likely to make a difference with more severe symptoms, more overall family dysfunction, and more diagnostic complexity.

Initiation of Counseling and Therapy

We recommend psychotherapy for any young person with moderate to severe symptoms meeting criteria for a mental health diagnosis or with mild symptoms that are persistent and dysfunctional enough to warrant the investment of the young person's time. There are exceptions to this broad generalization about when to recommend psychotherapy; for instance, even in severe cases of ADHD, the young person may be treated successfully with medications alone, but this is an exception to the rule. The specific preferred forms of psychotherapy differ by the type of disorder, so we encourage you to first identify the diagnosis and then consider the options we describe in Chapter 16, "Starting a Psychotherapy." Because many families avoid psychotherapy, you should learn their concerns and try to address them. For instance, "*You looked like you weren't very happy with the idea of working with a therapist. What comes to mind when you think about this?*"

One-on-one psychotherapy is only one source of outpatient services for young patients. Locally available support groups, crisis intervention services, parenting classes, social skills groups, family therapy, special education services, and speech therapists are just a few other examples. Because caregivers' own mental health difficulties may affect a young person's mental health disorders, coaching caregivers on their own appropriate use of psychotherapy may help a child or an adolescent. A clinician may use a question such as "*With everything going on, do you have someone in your corner who is there just to help or support you?*" Some primary care clinicians may provide young people with motivational interviewing techniques to reduce substance abuse behaviors or learn to provide coaching on relaxation training or other cognitive-behavioral techniques during their own follow-up appointments.

Appropriate Prescription of Medications

Primary care clinicians often feel pressured to prescribe right away, in part because the proverbial prescription pad is one of the few immediately available treatment tools. This can be quite appropriate when the diagnosis is clear, significant symptoms are present, an evidence-supported medication option is available, and the clinician has discussed the risks and benefits of medication with the family. We otherwise advise resisting immediately writing a prescription.

A near-universal recommendation when prescribing psychiatric medications to children is that some form of psychosocial intervention—therapy or changes in the child's environment—should accompany their use. Other prescribing principles to keep in mind include starting with low doses and increasing them slowly over time ("start low, go slow") and changing only one medication at a time to avoid outcomes confusion.

Here are our summary suggestions for a primary care approach to child mental health treatment:

- Instill appropriate hope, even in the initial interview.
- Form a therapeutic alliance with the young person and their caregivers.
- Use rating scales to help gather more clinical information, but be aware of their limitations.
- Ask for collateral information from other informants to help ensure a correct diagnosis.
- Interview adolescents alone to obtain a more complete history, especially for internalizing disorders.
- Note the child's behavior and interactions in the office, which supply much of your child mental status examination findings.
- For an initial brief assessment, make only a provisional DSM-5-TR unspecified diagnosis.
- Expect to use more than one appointment to refine your diagnoses with time-limited evaluations.
- Coach the family on pursuing their next best steps in care while screening for any barriers to address.
- For mild conditions, start with self-help approaches, bibliotherapy, and school interventions.
- Consider referring to specialist care anyone who is more seriously ill or not improving.
- Use psychosocial interventions, such as psychotherapy, in most scenarios.
- If symptoms are moderate to severe, consider starting medication management with an evidence-supported strategy.
- Use local specialists for support, to provide counseling, and to manage your more challenging patients.
- Schedule a follow-up appointment, even if patients are referred to specialty care.

Common Ages for Disorder Presentations

As we assess young people, we find it helpful to remember a maxim of clinical practice: "When you hear hoofbeats, think horses, not zebras." We find it easier to detect psychiatric conditions in young people by recognizing the typical ages when different mental health conditions are likely to appear. For instance, you are unlikely to diagnose anorexia nervosa, bipolar disorder, or schizophrenia in a 4-year-old.

Still, there are few precise ages at which you should or should not ever consider a particular diagnosis. We can offer no firm rules. But we can offer two pieces of prudent advice:

1. Remember the adage "Common things are common." When you are seeing a 10-year-old, separation anxiety disorder is more likely than schizophrenia.
2. Consider that developmental delay can influence the age and appearance of a disorder. For instance, encopresis, which is rarely seen in teenagers, may be more likely in a 16-year-old with the approximate mental age of a 4-year-old.

We created Table 2–1 from a survey of U.S. national households regarding current or ever-assigned mental health diagnoses for youth. It can guide your diagnostic inquiries by highlighting how common certain types of diagnoses may be (granted, family-reported diagnosis rates are not equivalent for all groups worldwide). You may notice, for instance, that anxiety problems are significantly more common than depression in child health.

According to data from the National Comorbidity Survey (Merikangas et al. 2010), anxiety disorders have a much earlier age at onset than many clinicians realize. Half of individuals who develop an anxiety disorder have symptom onset by age 6, half of those with behavior disorders have onset by age 11, and half of those with mood disorders have onset by age 13 (among adolescents who have a mental health diagnosis).

As children age, some conditions, such as encopresis and oppositional defiant disorder, become less likely, whereas conditions such as bipolar disorder and schizophrenia become more likely. We created Table 2–2, which lists diagnoses that are more likely to appear in different age cohorts of children, to reflect this overall difference in presentations. Overall, we can say that diagnosable mental health conditions increase with age. We advise against diagnosing personality disorders until at least late adolescence because, by definition, a child's personality develops and changes more actively than does an adult's personality.

TABLE 2–1. General frequencies of child disorders, per U.S. National Household Surveys of Child Health

Disorder	Occurrence	Frequency
ADHD (ages 3–17)	Ever told had disorder	9.8%
	Currently have disorder	8.7%
Behavior or conduct disorder (ages 3–17)	Ever told had disorder	8.9%
	Currently have disorder	7.0%
Anxiety (ages 3–17)	Ever told had disorder	9.4%
	Currently have disorder	7.8%
Depression (ages 3–17)	Ever told had disorder	4.4%
	Currently have disorder	3.4%
Autism spectrum disorder (ages 3–17)	Ever told had disorder	3.1%
	Currently have disorder	2.9%
Substance use disorder (ages 12–17)	In past year	4.1%

Source. Bitsko et al. 2022.

Age-Based Behavioral Health Screening

Knowing when different mental and behavioral health disorders typically appear in young people can help your diagnostic process. Any screening test or diagnostic inquiry has more positive predictive value the higher the overall prevalence of the condition being investigated. On the basis of prevalence rates and our own clinical experiences, the following are our

TABLE 2–2. Selected DSM-5-TR disorders to be considered at different ages

Preschool (2–5 years)	School age (6–12 years)	Adolescence (13–17 years)
ADHD (age ≥3, if severe)	ADHD	ADHD
Autism spectrum disorder	Adjustment disorder	Adjustment disorder
Communication disorders	Conduct disorder	Anorexia nervosa
Encopresis	Disruptive mood dysregulation disorder	Bipolar disorders
Intellectual disability (intellectual developmental disorder)	Encopresis	Bulimia nervosa
Oppositional defiant disorder	Insomnia disorder and parasomnias	Conduct disorder
Selective mutism	Intellectual disability (intellectual developmental disorder)	Generalized anxiety disorder
Separation anxiety disorder	Major depressive disorder	Insomnia disorder
Specific phobia	OCD	Intellectual disability (intellectual developmental disorder)
	Oppositional defiant disorder	Major depressive disorder
	PTSD	OCD
	Social anxiety disorder	Obstructive sleep apnea hypopnea
	Somatic symptom disorder	Oppositional defiant disorder
	Specific learning disorder	Panic disorder
	Specific phobia	Persistent depressive disorder
	Tourette's disorder (tics)	PTSD
	Trichotillomania (hair-picking disorder)	Schizophrenia
		Social anxiety disorder
		Somatic symptom disorder
		Specific learning disorder
		Specific phobia
		Substance use disorders
		Tourette's disorder (tics)
		Trichotillomania (hair-picking disorder)

Source. American Psychiatric Association 2022.

suggestions for routine consideration in your differential diagnosis at different age ranges.

Ages 0–5: Developmental impairments and problems with disruptive behavior are the predominant issues at these ages. General screening rating scales to consider at these ages include general developmental assessments, autism spectrum screens, and measures of social-emotional learning.

Ages 6–12: ADHD and disruptive, impulse-control, and conduct disorders; intellectual disabilities; anxiety disorders; and mood disorders predominate at these ages. General screening rating scales to consider at these ages include ADHD symptom rating scales, anxiety rating scales, and depression and autism spectrum measures.

Ages 13–18: Major depressive disorder, anxiety disorders, PTSD, eating disorders, ADHD, substance use disorder, and conduct disorder predominate at these ages. General screening rating scales to consider at these ages include ADHD symptom rating scales, anxiety rating scales, and depression rating scales.

Chapter 3

Engaging a Young Person Experiencing a Mental Health Crisis

Mental and behavioral health care for youth cannot always occur in calm situations. Sometimes a crisis requires an immediate response.

The first thing a clinician can do in any crisis is to center themselves. Maintaining the calmest state possible diminishes unconscious projections that negatively influence the distressing circumstances of a young patient. For youth and their caregivers who are on edge, a crisis can escalate further in the presence of a clinician who inadvertently expresses their own fears, frustrations, or even anger that a particular situation invokes. In contrast, a clinician who projects a sense of calm while working with a youth and family experiencing a crisis while speaking in a soft and slow voice typically helps defuse the crisis.

Mental health crises among youth can arise for many different reasons. Here we discuss how to approach the two most frequent mental health crisis concerns for youth: 1) suicidality and self-harm and 2) aggression.

Suicidality and Self-Harm

Youth suicidality is tragically common. In a 2019 self-report survey of U.S. adolescents in secondary school, around 18.8% of respondents had seriously considered attempting suicide in the past year, 15.7% had made a suicide plan, and 8.9% reported having attempted suicide, but only 2.5% reported seeking medical treatment for an attempt (Ivey-Stephenson et al. 2020). Indeed, very few young people experiencing suicidality are ever admitted to psychiatric hospitals. In one fashion or another, the vast majority of suicidality crises are handled in the community. Some youth never report their crises and suicidality to clinicians, either keeping their distress to themselves or seeking support from their families, friends, and community figures.

When youth do present to clinicians for support, we recommend starting with broad questions such as "*In the past few weeks, have you ever wished that you were dead?*" or "*In the past few weeks, have you been having thoughts about hurting yourself?*" If you get positive-sounding responses or nonverbal cues that this could be an area of difficulty for the patient, get more specific with follow-up questions such as "*In the past few weeks, have you thought about killing yourself? ...Are you having thoughts about killing yourself right now?*"

To make this process more straightforward for non–mental health specialists or to provide a standard procedure, some initial screening questions for suicidality like these have been summarized into a brief questionnaire called the Ask Suicide-Screening Questions (ASQ) tool, made available online by the National Institute of Mental Health (Table 3–1). "No" answers to the first four verbal screening items on the ASQ indicate a negative screen, with no need to then ask the final question. If a person answers affirmatively on item 5 of the ASQ, they need further evaluation, but an evaluator's overall clinical judgment always supersedes the specific item responses on the ASQ; performing a risk assessment is not just filling out a checklist. When formally assessing suicide risk, a clinician should interview the patient rather than relying on a self-questionnaire.

Assessing the overall safety of someone with suicidal thoughts requires understanding their situation in more detail because not everyone who has experienced suicidal thoughts needs to be referred for psychiatric hospitalization, the most intensive level of care. We think of this process as obtaining and recording enough clinical information such that any reasonable person would be able to weigh that same information and reach a similar conclusion about the patient's immediate safety needs.

To do a safety assessment, a clinician asks the youth questions about their thoughts, plans, past behaviors, current symptoms, and social supports. The secret to getting such information from a youth who is reluctant to engage is projecting a genuine desire to hear what things are like for them in their world. Your conversational style can be very much your

TABLE 3–1. Interview items from the Ask Suicide-Screening Questions (ASQ) tool

	Yes	No
1. In the past few weeks, have you wished you were dead?		
2. In the past few weeks, have you felt that you or your family would be better off if you were dead?		
3. In the past week, have you been having thoughts about killing yourself?		
4. Have you ever tried to kill yourself? (if so, when and how)		
(if yes to any of the above, ask the item below)		
5. Are you having thoughts of killing yourself right now?		

Source. National Institute of Mental Health 2024.

own, if you show genuine interest and give them time to talk. Adolescents are more likely to shut down in the presence of someone they feel is being fake, dismissive, or indifferent with them.

Toward the end of your assessment, you can also directly ask the youth "*Do you need help to keep yourself safe?*" to gain their overall self-assessment. A young person in a relatively low-risk situation may say they have suicidal thoughts but would never act on them because it would be against their religious beliefs to do so, say they have no specific plans for self-harm, and say they have good social supports. But another youth in a much higher risk situation may say they have very specific plans for self-harm via a highly lethal method (e.g., via a firearm or hanging) that they say is accessible to them, say they have nothing to live for, and say they have no active social supports in their life. It is that overall picture one is assessing for high or low risk.

A sample list of specific safety questions one could ask is available on the Brief Suicide Safety Assessment (BSSA), which is made available free online by the National Institute of Mental Health (see www.nimh.nih.gov/sites/default/files/documents/research/research-conducted-at-nimh/asq-toolkit-materials/youth-ed/bssa_ed_youth_asq_nimh_tool-kit.pdf). Examples of the BSSA suicidality screening questions, followed by current stressor and social support follow up questions, are listed below in the suggested order one might ask them of a patient:

- In the past few weeks, have you been thinking about killing yourself?
  - *If yes, ask* "How often?" "When was the last time?"
- Do you have a plan to kill yourself?
  - *If yes, ask* "What is your plan?"
  - *If no, ask* "If you were going to kill yourself, how would you do it?"
- Have you ever tried to hurt yourself?
- Have you ever tried to kill yourself?
  - *If yes, ask about how, when, and why and assess intent.*
- Is there a trusted adult you can talk to?
- Are there any conflicts at home that are hard to handle?
- Do you ever feel so much pressure at school that you can't take it anymore?
- Are you being bullied or picked on?
- Do you know anyone who has killed themselves or tried to kill themselves?
- What are some of the reasons you would *not* kill yourself?

A unique aspect of safety assessments with youth is communicating with caregivers. Although the primary part of a suicide safety interview is conducted with a youth alone, a collateral information interview with a caregiver joining the youth is important both to review the main aspects of their presenting history and to review safety concerns. First tell the patient that you will need to discuss safety concerns with their parent or legal guardian so that this will not come as a surprise.

When discussing youth-stated safety issues with a parent, first ask whether this information has already been shared with them. When a minor raises safety issues during the individual interview, it is a generally accepted practice to discuss these issues with a parent. The explicit goal of creating a safer environment for the youth can be a reason to breach the minor's individual confidentiality. It is often useful after a joint interview and safety discussion to ask the parent whether they would like to share anything in private—sometimes parents withhold very important information in front of their child.

The range of appropriate responses to a crisis involving suicidal thoughts in youth is very broad. For instance, less severe presentations could be responded to with recommendations for outpatient counseling and general home safety planning, such as increasing monitoring, removing easy access to lethal means of self-harm from the home, and planning whom to contact in a future crisis. Resources such as rapid access crisis appointments, home visit crisis services where they are available, or more frequent contacts with a current counselor can help to manage higher-risk situations in an outpatient environment. Inpatient hospitalization can be very helpful for keeping a youth safe during an acute crisis, although the overall benefits retrospectively reported by young patients posthospitalization vary.

In some cases a young patient may present with a self-harm-oriented crisis but deny any active suicidal thoughts or plans. It is important to clarify this difference if it exists with the youth and then be able to ensure that their caregiver understands the situation as well. Young people who are using self-harm as their coping mechanism are clearly struggling and in need of support. They also need to learn to use alternative coping strategies other than self-harm. At a minimum, such youth can be advised to engage further with outpatient counseling following their crisis.

We have intentionally not mentioned medications as one of the ways to respond to a suicidality crisis. Although antidepressant medications may yield benefits for some youth who have depressive disorders, if they do so it is a delayed response and not the means of rapidly resolving any suicidality crisis. The focus of the crisis response should instead be placed on counseling, social supports, and reducing access to lethal means.

Aggression

Another very common youth crisis presentation is aggression. Indeed, when preadolescent children are brought to an emergency department for a mental health concern, aggression is typically the primary concern (Tolliver et al. 2022). Aggression is a rather pan-diagnostic problem, in that youth with many different mental health disorders (or even without an underlying mental health disorder) can present with an aggression crisis. Typically, aggression happens when a young person has a self-perceived vital want or need that they feel cannot be achieved through nonforceful means. The triggering event for the aggression need not be something that others would perceive as a vital desire, such as a parent imposing a limit on their screen time.

Youth with limited language skills have a more difficult time navigating their place in the world and addressing their wants and needs. Parents of young children recognize this, in that preschool-age children often use aggression to get things they want, such as yelling "Mine!" while pulling a toy out of the hands of another child. Tantrums are also a very common early form of verbally or physically aggressive behavior when young children struggle to get something from their caregivers. During typical development, children usually learn to use their words instead to negotiate to get their needs met.

This typical developmental process away from the use of aggression can go awry for several reasons, such as when there are significant developmental (e.g., communication) delays, when children experience aggression by adults as a normalized action, or when children learn that tantrum-equivalent behaviors continue to work better for them than other strategies of getting what they want. This is why youth being brought to an emergency department setting for aggression crises are commonly found to have developmental impairments such as autism spectrum disorder, to have a history of significant past trauma exposures, or to have a long history of oppositional behavior patterns at home.

The clinician should think about how the child's aggression may be serving as a form of primitive communication in terms of theorizing about the etiology of the aggression. However, many other mental health disorders can contribute to a child having an irritable mood or can create conditions in which an aggressive outburst is more likely to occur. The differential diagnosis of possible underlying conditions causing irritability or more rapid aggression is broad and covers much of DSM-5-TR (American Psychiatric Association 2022). For instance, aggression is not a sign or symptom of OCD in DSM-5-TR, but if a child with severe OCD is stopped from performing one of their compulsive rituals, they may uncharacteristically lash out at the person stopping them.

When evaluating a youth who has recently had or is having an aggressive behavioral crisis, approach the situation with safety in mind. Keep yourself, other people, and the child safe during your evaluation process.

Safer mental health crisis evaluations can occur if you first have an opportunity to prepare the environment where the assessment will occur. You can simplify the space by removing distracting objects, items that pose a potential safety risk (e.g., any needles that might be present in an emergency department), and dangerous objects that can be thrown or broken and should address potential building hazards (e.g., avoid interviews in isolated settings). When working with patients who are known to be aggressive, evaluators should try to position themselves on the same side of the room as the door (for an easy exit if necessary) and to have a clear means of requesting assistance if needed.

There is an important distinction to be made between identifying youth behaviors that are *upsetting* versus behaviors that are *unsafe*. An aggressively yelling child is not in the same situation as a child who is physically attacking others. Differentiate between when a behavior is so unsafe that a highly restrictive intervention is required and when children can safely express their anger without being restricted. In an emergency department, for instance, something like a restraint or an involuntarily injected medication would not be appropriate for a child exhibiting upsetting behaviors such as verbally expressing anger at their overall circumstances. Many children who present to hospitals in aggressive crises have a history of past trauma, and we desire to avoid restraining these children because it can be retraumatizing.

Usually, but not always, physical aggression occurs after other recognizable steps along the way toward an aggressive act. In this process you might expect that verbal agitation (raised voice, yelling) would come before physical agitation (pacing or aggression toward objects), before verbal threats (threat of consequences if their demands are not met), before physical threats (raised fist, throwing of objects at a person), and before physical violence toward a person. Although it may be appropriate to deliver your usual calm and supportive listening and coaching to a child who is verbally or physically agitated, by the time the child reaches the level of making verbal or physical threats, a different approach is needed. In general, if a child is actively threatening, we would advise backing off and giving them space, asking for additional support as appropriate and available, and minimizing or stopping the verbal engagement until the child is calmer.

This mirrors, in a way, the common advice offered to parents of a young child having a tantrum—that talking to or bargaining with a child during a tantrum is unproductive. Instead, ignoring or walking away from the tantrum is essentially the best approach to getting the child to learn that their physical or verbal threat behaviors do not work in getting the child what they want. When they are calm again and communicative, the child sees that life can go on.

With circumstances arranged such that an interview with the child can be safely conducted, the diagnostic process can proceed as usual. We pay attention to what has happened before with other aggressive episodes, with a particular understanding of the sequence of events (with close attention to a parent-offered history) and what may have changed in the child's world to lead up to the presenting aggressive episode. For children with long-term medication plans, a crisis sometimes occurs with medication changes, so we would be sure to ask about this as well.

When youth have very limited verbal abilities, aggressive acts need to be investigated with their caregiver in terms of the behavior's potential function, in what would broadly be termed the ABCs of a functional analysis of behavior: What was happening before (Antecedents), during (Behavior), and right after (Consequences) the behavior that might explain why it occurred and therefore what might influence it to occur again in the future? This questioning process can lead to hypotheses about what triggers or perpetuates the aggression, which can lead to new intervention approach trials to see whether the aggressive behavior pattern changes (see Chapter 15, "Initiating Psychosocial Interventions," for more on functional analysis of behavior).

Parents or hospital staff often ask for a medication to be prescribed to treat aggression, but there is no simple response that would fit every situation. Acute, in-the-moment treatment of an irritable and aggressive mood state begins with talking and listening, not medication. The next step is problem-solving. In an emergency department, this can be something as concrete as addressing basic needs by bringing the child something to eat and drink.

The only FDA-approved medications for treating irritability in youth are risperidone and aripiprazole, but they are approved only in the context of an autism spectrum disorder. Aggressive mood states can often be acutely altered by the judicious administration of antihistamine (with some risk of paradoxic excitation), benzodiazepine (with some risk of worsening via disinhibition), and antipsychotic medications. If you decide to pursue medications, oral formulations should always be offered first, and both consent and assent should be sought. If necessary, these medications can be administered intramuscularly or, in very rare cases, intravenously, but such emergency use of involuntary medications should always be second-line treatment and conducted in accordance with local regulations and laws. Although it is sometimes necessary, the involuntary use of medication with a child or adolescent is always the clinically undesired path.

Finally, if a patient has an underlying DSM-5-TR diagnosis for which a medication is a recognized effective treatment, such as the use of a stimulant medication for ADHD, then this medication intervention should be included as an approach in their care plan. Pursuing evidence-based and person-centered treatment of any underlying conditions is one of the best ways to address recurrent aggression in a young person.

Postcrisis Planning for Caregivers

After a major crisis event with a young person, it helps to develop a prevention plan for future crises. The following is a list of tips you can provide parents for postcrisis planning in the home.

1. In the home environment, maintain a low-key atmosphere and keep up regular routines.
2. Follow typical house rules, but pick your battles. For example:
    -   If a child engages in aggressive or dangerous behaviors, intervene immediately.
    -   If a child is using oppositional words, you may be able to ignore those words.
3. Provide appropriate supervision until the crisis is resolved (i.e., always have an adult around).
4. Make a specific crisis prevention plan:
    -   Identify likely triggers for a crisis (such as an argument).
    -   Plan with the child what to do the next time the triggers occur (e.g., remove oneself from the situation

until feeling calm again, call a friend, engage in a distracting activity).

5. Encourage your child to attend school unless otherwise directed by a clinician.

6. Attend the next scheduled appointment with your clinician.

7. Administer medications as directed by the child's medical or psychiatric clinician.

8. Enter each day and evening with a plan for how time will be spent—this should help prevent boredom and arguments in the moment.

9. If there are self-harm risks, secure and lock up all medications and objects a child or an adolescent could use to hurt themselves, including the following:

- Sharp objects such as knives and razors
- Materials that can be used for strangulation attempts, such as belts, cords, ropes, and sheets
- Firearms and ammunition (these should be locked and kept in separate locations from each other)
- Medications of all family members, including all over-the-counter medicines

10. In the event of another crisis, do the following:

- Contact your health care provider.
- Call 911 to have your child transported to the nearest emergency department if you believe that the child, yourself, or another person is no longer safe because of their behavior.
- Use local and national crisis and suicide hotlines.

Chapter 4

Working Together on Common Clinical Concerns

Every child or adolescent is unique, but a handful of common concerns account for most of the reasons young people come to clinical attention. During training, a clinician learns to recognize these patterns of common problems. You see hundreds of children and adolescents, discuss them with clinical supervisors, and develop a subconscious ability to quickly recognize the ways in which a particular child resembles common patterns. For instance, you might quickly recognize a child's presentation pattern as typical of an uncomplicated adjustment to a new school rather than an episode of major depression. These subconscious patterns are a tremendous benefit to a clinician because they improve clinical efficacy and efficiency.

However, relying on experience to guide your current practice can cause at least two problems in the diagnostic process: failing to recognize that personal practice experience does not apply to all situations and neglecting the potential for assumption-based diagnostic mistakes. First, even seasoned clinicians make mistakes. We could assume that an adolescent has an ordinary case of situational unhappiness (such as an adjustment disorder) and then neglect to consider whether their social isolation is the result of abuse, major depression, or psychosis. Or we could assume that a child's inability to play well with others represents a neurodevelopmental disorder, so we neglect to ask about cultural expectations for interactive play in a family. Even an experienced clinician needs to remain curious about a particular patient, their family, and their cultural environment while being vigilant about making mistakes.

Second, most young people are evaluated and treated for mental illness by primary care clinicians with limited mental health training. These clinicians often have remarkable stores of clinical experience in caring for children and adolescents, but their specialized mental health training is often limited. A clinician whose training is not specialized for mental health can benefit from referencing prudent aids to decision-making.

The following sections, and their accompanying tables, are intended as general guides to how one might approach common clinical concerns as they might appear in practice. Each table identifies a common clinical concern, provides diagnostic categories to which the concern can be mapped, and suggests simple screening questions to guide clinical inquiry. We designed most questions to be asked of a young person. When a question is designed to be asked of a caregiver, we label it "for caregiver."

These are the common clinical concern categories we have organized for you in this chapter:

- Poor academic performance
- Developmental delay
- Disruptive or aggressive behavior
- Withdrawn or sad mood
- Irritable or labile mood
- Anxious or avoidant behavior
- Recurrent or excessive physical complaints
- Sleep problems
- Self-harm and suicidality
- Substance abuse
- Disturbed eating
- Postpartum maternal mental health

Poor Academic Performance

To succeed in a work environment, a person needs the ability to succeed, the desire to succeed, and an environment that enables success. Major life distractions or impairing illnesses can unfortunately derail a person who would otherwise find success. Although that simple description can be used to describe just about any adult workplace, the exact same points are true about children in school. School is where children and adolescents go to work.

When you see a child who is struggling to succeed in school, it is useful to think very broadly about what might be getting in their way (Table 4–1). Just like an adult who is hav-

TABLE 4–1. Screening questions for poor academic performance

	Suggested questions
First consider	
Abuse	*"Has anything or anyone made you feel uncomfortable or unsafe?"*
	(for caregiver) *"Has anything happened to your child that really shouldn't have happened?"*
Bullying	*"Have other kids been teasing you or making you feel afraid?"*
Sensory impairment	*"Have you ever noticed any trouble with your hearing or vision?"*
Common diagnostic possibilities	
ADHD	(for caregiver) *"Even when she wants to learn, is your child too inattentive or hyperactive to succeed?"*
Intellectual disability (intellectual developmental disorder)	(for caregiver) *"Have there always been problems with learning? Were there early delays in development, such as speech delays?"*
Specific learning disorder	*"Are any specific subjects or activities in school, such as reading, particularly difficult?"*
Mood or anxiety disorder	(for caregiver) *"Did poor school performance come after an anxious or depressive change?"*
Oppositional defiant disorder or conduct disorder	(for caregiver) *"Is your child simply refusing to do schoolwork?"*
Substance use disorder	*"Have you been using drugs or alcohol?"*

ing workplace difficulties, a young person may be having problems with 1) ability, 2) desire or effort, 3) the work environment, 4) a life distraction, or 5) an impairing mental health disorder or illness.

Ability challenges we consider right away to ensure we do not miss them. The most basic ability is sensing. Hearing and vision screens are easy to perform, and an intervention such as a hearing aid or a new pair of glasses can make a profound difference. Motor impairments, such as the physical inability to write or enunciate clearly, also can be managed effectively through physical, occupational, or speech therapy.

Intellectual disabilities, of course, greatly influence school success. You can determine whether a young child has fallen behind on developmental milestones by comparing their traits with a list of normal-range expectations (see Chapter 13, "Recognizing Developmental Red Flags," Table 13–1). Caregiver-completed developmental rating scale measures such as the Ages and Stages Questionnaires (ASQ) aid in this task, or you can simply ask a caregiver if they have any concerns about the child's speech, comprehension, or physical development. We would suspect an intellectual disability when the child has multiple areas of delay. IQ test scores provide helpful data, but impairments in adaptive life functioning also must be present for an intellectual disability diagnosis. Early intervention services or a local school district's special education program should be engaged as early as possible to improve outcomes when global developmental delay or an intellectual disability is suspected.

Specific learning disabilities are often detected much later than a general intellectual disability because they may not become apparent until school demands increase. The three overall categories of specific learning disabilities are reading, writing, and computation. The hallmark of a specific learning disability is that the child has an area of much poorer school performance than expected on the basis of the child's overall intellect and effort.

Desire or effort in school is about the motivation to achieve. A person with a low to average intellect but a strong motivation to achieve can have greater school success than someone with high intellect but low motivation to achieve. There is no quick fix for motivation problems. For parents seeking one, it can be helpful to clarify that there is certainly no pill that creates in children a motivation to achieve. For young children, motivation in school starts with healthy home relationships and regularly experienced positive parent-child time that fosters a desire within children to meet adult expectations. Positive experiences of working toward and reaching small goals in different areas of life further build a child's sense of competency and resilience. Clear and reasonable family expectations for a child's school achievement are also necessary. For older children, this desire to achieve ideally evolves into working hard in school because they want to please themselves rather than simply to please others.

The *work environment* affects performance because not every school and not every classroom suits every child. For instance, an easily distracted child will not do well in a loud and overcrowded classroom, and a child with a specific writing disability will not do well in a class that requires completing large volumes of daily written work. Asking about the class environment and the child's home workspace may identify these issues.

Life distractions prevent success by taking a child's mind off their schoolwork. Abuse, neglect, and bullying are the most important distractions for us to catch right away so that child protective services or school officials can intervene. Children may experience a decline in school performance because of family stressors such as parental separation or divorce or as a result of struggling with peer relationships. It is useful to ask, *"When you try to do your schoolwork but get distracted, what's on your mind?"*

Impairing mental health disorders or illnesses that are described in DSM-5-TR (American Psychiatric Association 2022) can create school problems. For instance, major depressive disorder, persistent depressive disorder, generalized anxiety disorder, obsessive-compulsive disorder (OCD), social anxiety disorder, oppositional defiant disorder, conduct disorder, substance use disorder, and posttraumatic stress disorder (PTSD) all negatively affect a child's school performance. Chronic medical diseases, especially when they result in chronic pain, also reduce the ability to focus on school.

Attention-deficit/hyperactivity disorder (ADHD) ranks at the top of mental disorders in terms of overall incidence (>5%) and common family requests for treatment. We look for ADHD if difficulties related to attention or hyperactivity can be traced back to the early elementary school years and are not readily attributed to any of the causes mentioned earlier. Attention problems with a relatively sudden onset are unlikely to be caused by ADHD. Another thing to look for is whether ADHD-like symptoms are present in multiple settings (such as both in school and at home). The good news is that by correctly identifying an impairing illness such as ADHD, you have an opportunity to treat and resolve the schooling problem.

Developmental Delay

A person's development from infancy to adulthood is amazing in its breadth and complexity. Because not every person develops at the same pace or acquires skills in the same order, detecting a significant developmental impairment may be challenging (Table 4–2). For instance, a child may learn to walk without ever crawling or may appear to have delayed speech at 18 months but advanced speech at 2 years. Fewer than half of the children with significant developmental delays are identified before they start school, which delays entry into treatment. Therefore, anything clinicians can do to help caregivers detect these problems can alter the trajectory of a child's life. A key function of health maintenance care in the first 5 years of life is to detect developmental impairments that would benefit from an intervention. Any parental concerns expressed about a child's speech, learning, sociability, or physical skills should open the proverbial door for further examination.

Development can be broken down into three broad categories: cognitive, motor, and social-emotional. *Cognitive development* refers to what most people think of as intelligence. Some measurable areas of cognition include problem-solving, language, memory, information processing, and attention. *Motor development* refers to the acquisition of gross motor (e.g., running, throwing) and fine motor (e.g., pincer grasp, drawing) physical motion skills. *Social-emotional development* refers to the acquisition of the ability to interact with others and manage the emotions of social interactions.

Because there is a very wide range of what can be considered typical development, we look for developmental markers that are far enough outside the norm to justify referral for developmental assessments or interventions. When parents express that they already have concerns about a specific area of their child's development, we will likely find a need for a developmental assessment referral. Speech therapists can help with suspected communication delays, physical therapists can help with suspected motor skill delays, and special education–sponsored preschools can help with suspected socialization and general learning skill delays. All children with significant developmental delays should be referred to early intervention services.

Detecting autism spectrum disorder before a child reaches age 3 years is aided by recognizing certain red flags

TABLE 4–2. Screening questions for developmental delay

	Suggested questions for caregiver
First consider	
Neurodegenerative conditions	*"Has your child lost any previously acquired skills or abilities?"*
Sensory impairment	*"Have you ever noticed any trouble with your child's hearing or vision?"*
Common diagnostic possibilities	
Autism spectrum disorder	*"Does your child smile in response to your smile? Did your child respond to their own name before age 1? Does your child have restricted interests or behaviors?"*
Communication disorder	*"Does your child have problems with stuttering or with understanding words?"*
Fragile X syndrome	*"Does your child have siblings or relatives on the mother's side of the family with intellectual impairment?"*
Intellectual disability (intellectual developmental disorder) or global developmental delay	*"Was your child slow to develop speech and physical skills? Does your child have a harder time learning new things than other children?"*
Neurobehavioral disorder associated with prenatal alcohol exposure	*"What can you tell me about alcohol use during pregnancy? Has your child had difficulty regulating their mood or impulses?"*

in social-emotional development. These include not smiling in response to being smiled at, not making eye contact, not sharing attention with others, not responding to their own name by age 1 year, poor social interest, and a lack of interest in other children. Socially focused interventions that foster communication as early as possible are a cornerstone of autism care.

Every child with developmental impairment should be screened for hearing or vision impairments because sensory impairments can worsen or even cause developmental impairments. Another reason to perform early sensory assessments is that hearing and vision impairments can be relatively easy to treat.

A developmental impairment rarely worsens over time, so when we find any loss of previously acquired skills, we broaden our search for an etiology to include medical causes. Hypothyroidism, phenylketonuria, and recurrent seizures are some of the many medical causes of regressing development.

We recommend considering genetic testing if the clinical pattern might fit a genetic disorder for either prognosis purposes or general family information purposes (sharing the likelihood or not of similar impairments with future offspring). For instance, fragile X testing could be particularly pertinent if other family members have intellectual disability. If no specific genetic disorder is suspected, the yield of genetic testing is reduced. Developmental disorder laboratory tests for fragile X and chromosome microarray should be ordered only after pretest counseling is provided to families. Family risks from genetic testing include finding a mutation of unknown significance that creates more anxiety than answers or learning something the family did not wish to learn, such as misattributed paternity or a pessimistic prognosis that lowers current quality of life.

Diagnosing a child with neurobehavioral disorder associated with prenatal alcohol exposure, which is included in Section III of DSM-5-TR, can present a challenge to your therapeutic alliance with caregivers because it implies blame for some of a child's problems on the mother's behaviors during pregnancy. Characteristic facial features (thin upper lip, smooth philtrum, short palpebral fissure length) might be present, but their absence does not rule out the diagnosis. Because these children have a unique prognosis, it is worth exploring this possibility in a blame-free fashion.

In Chapter 13, we further review developmental milestones and discuss developmental red flags, signs that need further evaluation, ideally through specialized developmental assessments.

Disruptive or Aggressive Behavior

When we see a young person who is aggressive or disruptive, we receive their behavior as a form of communication. A child who is unable to effectively communicate verbally may use behaviors instead, such as lashing out at a peer who has just taken their toy. Hunger, pain, sadness, fear, and frustration are just a few examples of distress that may turn into tantrums, disruptive behavior, or aggression. For instance, if you can identify that hunger leads to a tantrum in a nonverbal child, the child can be coached to point at a picture of food to communicate hunger and get something to eat (this is known as a *picture exchange system*).

A *functional analysis of behavior* is an overall approach that helps with most aggression problems in childhood. In a functional analysis, you identify the character, timing, frequency, and duration of at least a few incidents of disruptive, aggressive behavior in great detail. Predisposing, precipitating, and perpetuating influences on behavior can be elicited by asking a series of questions, such as *"Tell me about the last time this happened. What was happening right before? How had that day been going overall? What did you do while the behavior was happening? What happened right afterward?"*

What you often discover from the unedited details of two or three incidents is that the aggressive and disruptive behaviors begin to make a lot more sense. Examples include tantrums inadvertently being rewarded with treats because caregivers want the child to stop in the moment or aggression that allows a child to successfully escape aversive situations.

Different DSM-5-TR disorders may be suggested by circumstances of the child's disruptive behaviors (Table 4–3). Children with PTSD may become disruptive when situations remind them of past negative events. Children with a learning disorder may be disruptive when struggling at school or working on homework. A child with ADHD may have nearly continuous disruptive hyperactivity that is not situational or vindictive. A child with social anxiety disorder or autism spectrum disorder may show disruptive behavior when pushed to engage in social situations. A child who has been bullied at school may suddenly develop disruptive, lashing-out behavior or become resistant to going to school. In summary, identifying the overall pattern and context of behaviors is key to the diagnostic process.

It is relatively easy to identify oppositional defiant disorder, a diagnosis describing pervasively negativistic and defiant behavior toward authority figures that is developmentally inappropriate (i.e., not just the terrible twos) and that lasts for more than 6 months. The real challenge is knowing what to do about it.

Oppositional defiant disorder has a complex, multifactorial etiology. In simple terms, we find it useful to think of this

TABLE 4–3. Screening questions for disruptive or aggressive behavior

	Suggested screening questions
First consider	
Abuse	"Has anything or anyone made you feel uncomfortable or unsafe?"
	(for caregiver) "Has anything happened to your child that really shouldn't have happened?"
Bullying	"Have other kids been teasing you or making you feel afraid?"
Safety	"Have you been thinking about or planning to hurt anyone?"
Common diagnostic possibilities	
ADHD	(for caregiver) "Does your child consistently have trouble paying attention, or is she hyperactive or disruptive?"
Communication disorder	(for caregiver) "Is your child aggressive when he has needs he cannot communicate?"
Conduct disorder	(for caregiver) "Has your child been committing serious violations of rules and the rights of others for more than a year?"
Oppositional defiant disorder	(for caregiver) "Has your child been unusually defiant and oppositional for more than 6 months?"
PTSD	(for caregiver) "Does your child's disruptive behavior primarily occur after reminders or memories of past trauma?"

disorder as representing a mismatch in fit between a child's inherent traits or temperament and how their caregivers and authority figures respond to them. Communicating to caregivers that they share responsibility with their child for the negative behavior patterns in oppositional defiant disorder without this being perceived as blaming them for the problem is a tricky balance. One way to do this is to characterize the child's personality or biology as demanding more than usual from parents, so more highly skilled parenting strategies are needed to respond to the resulting behavior patterns. Empathy for the challenge parents face goes a long way here.

Conduct disorder is a similar, but more concerning, version of defiant, aggressive behavior that has a greater risk of continuing into adulthood. Conduct disorder should be suspected when a child is committing serious violations of the rights of others, such as stealing, initiating fights, using a weapon to threaten others, destroying property, or running away from home.

Successful management of oppositional defiant disorder and conduct disorder requires motivating authority figures in a child's environment to make changes in how they interact with the child. The traditional one-on-one psychotherapy approach is rarely sufficient. Behavior management training is the best overall strategy for treating both oppositional defiant disorder and conduct disorder. There are many types of behavior management training, but they all share a focus on coaching parents and caregivers to more skillfully set limits and expectations for the child and a focus on the child and parents regularly spending positive time together, thus providing opportunities for the child to experience praise. Historically, this approach was referred to as *parent training*, but we think that term should be discarded for unnecessarily assigning fault to the parents, which reduces the therapeutic alliance and motivation for change. The more severe the youth's symptoms, the more community inclusive the behavior management approach should be, such as how multisystemic therapy also engages nonparental authority figures in the community for patients with conduct disorder.

Medications are generally not the preferred treatment for disruptive or aggressive behavior. However, if the child has a specific diagnosis that is known to be responsive to medication, such as ADHD or major depressive disorder, then medication treatment typically will also improve disruptive or aggressive behavior. No medications are independently indicated for the treatment of oppositional defiant disorder or conduct disorder; the best treatment is via coaching and supporting the child's authority figures. However, if a disruptive or aggressive problem is highly impairing and other appropriate interventions have been tried and have failed, then a nonspecific medication to diminish maladaptive or impulsive aggression may be considered. If this is done, we recommend a trial of clonidine or guanfacine first because if it is helpful, use of these medications presents few long-term medical risks. Second-generation antipsychotics, often starting with risperidone, can reduce aggression, but antipsychotics have more significant adverse effects, especially adverse metabolic effects, and should be reserved for the most severe scenarios after parent-training interventions have been tried (Loy et al. 2017).

Withdrawn or Sad Mood

When a young person presents as withdrawn, anhedonic, or sad (Table 4–4), we always assess for the presence of a major depressive episode. Two or more weeks of depressed or irritable mood, along with multiple neurovegetative symptoms (decreased energy, concentration, interest, or physical activity; thoughts of self-harm; changes in appetite or sleep; and feelings of guilt or worthlessness), would suggest a major depressive episode. In contrast, persistent depressive disorder is essentially a low-grade depression that has been present for more than a year in a child without relief for more than 2 months during that time. If the sad mood was triggered by a stressful event within the past 3 months and neither major depression nor persistent depressive disorder is diagnosable, an adjustment disorder with depressed mood may be present.

Regardless of whether or not a withdrawn or sad child has an active mood disorder, routinely asking about self-harm risks is important. Adolescents may see even a single disappointment—such as a relationship breakup—as so catastrophic that they feel suicidal or begin to hurt themselves. This means that as clinicians we must ask about suicidal thoughts and self-harm urges even if we believe that a young person is experiencing only a time-limited adjustment disorder. With practice, asking about suicidality and self-harm comes as naturally as asking any other question. Remember: asking about suicidal thoughts does not create a risk of self-harm, but instead reduces risks by showing you care.

Although a medically induced depression is uncommon in a young person, all clinicians must be alert to the possibility. For instance, testing for hypothyroidism is reasonable if a patient experienced a physical symptom such as fatigue before mood changes developed. Because anemia can occur in young people, a complete blood count should be considered

TABLE 4–4. Screening questions for withdrawn or sad mood

	Suggested questions
First consider	
Abuse	*"Has anything or anyone made you feel uncomfortable or unsafe?"*
	(for caregiver) *"Has anything happened to your child that really shouldn't have happened?"*
Bullying	*"Have other kids been teasing you or making you feel afraid?"*
Medical conditions (anemia, hypothyroidism)	*"Did all of your symptoms seem to start with fatigue?"*
Self-harm	*"Have you been thinking about hurting yourself? Have you ever hurt yourself or attempted suicide? Do you have any plans to hurt yourself?"*
Common diagnostic possibilities	
Adjustment disorder with depressed mood	*"Did your sad or down mood start right after a stressful event in the past few months?"*
Bipolar disorder	*"Has there ever been a period of multiple days in a row when you were the opposite of depressed, with very high energy and little need for sleep? If so, can you tell me more about that time?"*
Major depressive disorder	*"Have you felt really down, depressed, or uninterested in things you used to enjoy for more than 2 weeks?"*
Persistent depressive disorder	*"Have you been sad or gloomy most days of the week for more than a year?"*
Substance use disorder	*"Have you been using drugs or alcohol?"*

to assess its presence in a patient who is fatigued. Iatrogenic origins of depression should be considered as well, such as when a child starting β-blockers or isotretinoin subsequently experiences dysphoria.

Recurrent substance abuse can cause an adolescent to appear depressed. Because we find that adolescents typically assert that they see their substance use as helping their mood, establishing a timeline of what came first may help you convince your patient to discontinue the substance at least temporarily and find out how they feel after a few weeks or more of being substance free.

Bipolar disorder is relatively uncommon in children but should be considered. To detect the possibility of bipolar depression, we ask caregivers if the child has ever had a history of discrete mood elevation and energy increase of multiple days' duration with accompanying manic symptoms (e.g., racing thoughts or speech, unusual risk-taking, decreased need for sleep). Note that the presence of an irritable mood is not a reliable indicator of bipolar disorder in children. If you suspect that a young person with a withdrawn or sad mood has bipolar disorder, monotherapy with antidepressants should be avoided because of their risk for inducing a manic episode.

Every child with a moderate to severe depressive disorder should be referred for an evidence-based psychotherapy, such as cognitive-behavioral therapy (CBT) or interpersonal therapy. Because not every family will be motivated to use psychotherapy, we inform families about the treatment value of psychotherapy, telling them that psychotherapy is the most effective strategy available to reduce the risk of suicidality. Caregivers of a young person can also take the safety steps of restricting impulsive access to firearms and dangerous pills and maintaining increased awareness and monitoring. In the presence of active suicide plans or the inability to maintain immediate safety, clinicians should consider admission to a crisis stabilization unit, day treatment program, or psychiatric inpatient treatment. Families also can help the child by promoting behavioral activation treatment for depression at home through scheduling desirable exercise and social activities.

The current view on use of selective serotonin reuptake inhibitors (SSRIs) to treat depression is that some young patients might experience an increase in suicidal thoughts during the first few months of SSRI use, but most do not, and overall, the benefits of their use outweigh potential risks for a moderate to severe depression. A prudent clinician will warn patients about the possible risk, stay connected with patients and caregivers after the initial prescription, inquire specifically at least twice in the first month of use about increased irritability or suicidal thoughts, and strongly consider stopping the medication if suicidal ideation occurs or irritability increases (Murphy et al. 2021).

Because of its larger evidence base indicating benefits in young people, fluoxetine is typically considered the first-line medicine for adolescent major depressive disorder. Second-line SSRI choices based on the evidence include sertraline and escitalopram or citalopram. Usual starting doses for treating adolescent depression are 10 mg for fluoxetine, 25–50 mg for sertraline, 10 mg for citalopram, and 5 mg for escitalopram; about half of these amounts are used in preadolescents. Doses should be increased after 4–6 weeks if the medications are well tolerated but have insufficient benefits. SSRIs are most effective when used in combination with psychotherapy, which is another reason to promote the family's engagement with psychotherapy. Persistent depressive disorder is treated with the same medications, but response is notably slower and less reliable (Schramm et al. 2020).

Irritable or Labile Mood

A young person may experience an irritable or labile mood for many different reasons (Table 4–5). Several mental disorders—bipolar disorders, depressive disorders, anxiety disorders, PTSD, and oppositional defiant disorder—should be considered because irritability can be a symptom of a mental disorder. It also can be a symptom of substance abuse, a reaction to challenging life situations or maltreatment, or a normal variation in mood. When irritability is the primary complaint, we counsel a broad search for clues as to why.

Unfortunately, there has been a misdiagnosis problem in which chronically irritable, labile moods in children have been interpreted as pathognomonic of a childhood bipolar disorder. This was usually incorrect, in that few (if any) chronically irritable children were later found to have bipolar disorder as young adults (Birmaher et al. 2014). Unless a child has a multiday duration of manic symptoms occurring during a discrete episode that represents a break from their baseline functioning, we counsel against diagnosing bipolar disorder in children and adolescents.

TABLE 4–5. Screening questions for irritable or labile mood

	Suggested questions
First consider	
Abuse	*"Has anything or anyone made you feel uncomfortable or unsafe?"*
	(for caregiver) *"Has anything happened to your child that really shouldn't have happened?"*
Substance abuse	*"Have you been using drugs or alcohol?"*
Suicidality	*"Have you had thoughts about hurting yourself?"*
Common diagnostic possibilities	
Bipolar disorder	*"Has there ever been a period of multiple days in a row when you were the opposite of depressed, with super high energy and little need for sleep? If so, can you tell me more about that time?"*
Disruptive mood dysregulation disorder	(for caregiver) *"Has your child had severe and persistent irritability along with frequent temper outbursts?"*
Major depressive disorder	*"Have you felt really down, depressed, or uninterested in things you used to enjoy for more than 2 weeks?"*
Oppositional defiant disorder	(for caregiver) *"Has your child been unusually defiant and oppositional for more than 6 months?"*
PTSD	(for caregiver) *"Does the irritability or moodiness worsen after reminders or memories of past trauma?"*

In part because of the recognition that a diagnosis was required to better characterize children with life dysfunction due to chronically irritable and dysphoric moods (who used to be mislabeled *bipolar*), a new diagnosis was created. Disruptive mood dysregulation disorder was added to DSM-5 to describe children who have more than a year of significant daily dysphoric mood symptoms and temper outbursts three or more times a week that are not better explained by other conditions. Practically speaking, it can be useful to think of disruptive mood dysregulation disorder as a variant of oppositional defiant disorder in which mood and irritability symptoms predominate and typically last for a period of a few years.

Even if a young person's irritability cannot ultimately be traced to a specific diagnosis with a known treatment, a generalized approach to managing irritable moods can still be helpful. We recommend enhancing family supports and providing behavior management training as appropriate care for most types of irritable mood. Creating calm, consistent, and caring limits and expectations within the household will typically improve behavior problems and irritability from a wide variety of causes.

Families with significant internal conflict can benefit from family therapy or from caregivers seeking their own individual supports. You may be able to motivate parents who report feeling exasperated with a child by using the analogy of putting your own mask on first, as with airline travel. An unnurtured parent who receives individual supports or professional help may greatly improve interactions with their child. For those children who are found to lack positive experiences with their caregivers, creating opportunities for praise and positive attention is a key to successful treatment.

One-on-one counseling therapy is indicated for all mood disorders and anxiety-related conditions (including PTSD) with an irritability component. Medication is never indicated for irritable mood without a specific diagnosis.

Anxious or Avoidant Behavior

When a child is struggling with being worried or anxious, we first check whether something in the child's world is directly causing this feeling. Anxiety from being bullied, from experiencing a major traumatic event, or from living in an abusive household should appropriately generate self-protective avoidance behaviors. Only after we know that no realistic and ongoing threat to the child exists and have determined that the child's anxiety causes significant life dysfunction do we consider an anxiety disorder diagnosis (Table 4–6).

Children have worries during typical development, such as fears of strangers, separation, injury, or failure. Learning

TABLE 4–6. Screening questions for anxious or avoidant behavior

Suggested questions

First consider

Abuse — "Has anything or anyone made you feel uncomfortable or unsafe?"

(for caregiver) "Has anything happened to your child that really shouldn't have happened?"

Bullying — "Have other kids been teasing you or making you feel afraid?"

Self-harm — "When you feel overwhelmed, do you think about hurting yourself?"

Trauma — "Have you been hurt recently or been in any accidents?"

Common diagnostic possibilities

Generalized anxiety disorder — "Do you feel tense, restless, or worried most of the time? Do these worries affect your sleep or performance at school?"

OCD — "Do you frequently have unwanted thoughts, images, or urges in your mind? Do you check or clean things to avoid those unwanted thoughts?"

Panic disorder — "Do you get sudden surges of fear that make your body feel shaky or your heart race? Do you change what you do to avoid having a panic experience?"

PTSD — "Do you startle easily or have frequent nightmares? Do you avoid reminders of traumatic events in your past?"

(for caregiver) "Does the irritability or moodiness worsen after reminders or memories of past trauma?"

Separation anxiety disorder — "Is it hard to leave your house or hard to leave your mom or dad because of worries?"

Specific phobia — "Is there something in particular or a situation that makes you immediately afraid?"

how to cope with anxious feelings by facing them directly is an important developmental task that, once mastered, enables future achievements. Parental anxiety may interfere with this process if it reinforces a child's fears or encourages avoidance behavior. For instance, inadvertent parental reinforcement of normal separation anxiety, such as allowing the child to stay home from school as a means of reassurance in response to separation fears, may turn this problem into a disorder over time unless the parent is taught more helpful strategies.

Children who feel anxious often struggle to find words to express how they feel. A child reporting stomachache, nausea, chest pain, fatigue, or headache may be functionally disclosing that they feel anxious, but through a biological mechanism such as their autonomic nerves altering intestinal motility or arterial smooth muscle tone. In fact, the chief complaint of children and adolescents seeking mental health treatment in primary care settings is often a physical ailment. When listening alertly for any meaning behind a physical ailment, clinicians should think about timing. Severe stomach cramps before attending school or headaches before performing in a sporting event will help you identify anxiety disorders.

Common anxiety disorders in children include generalized anxiety disorder, panic disorder, specific phobia, and separation anxiety disorder. These conditions could appear in a developmental trajectory, such as separation anxiety disorder during the elementary school years being replaced by specific phobias in middle school and then a generalized anxiety disorder in the adolescent years. For some children, their anxiety trait persists, but the expressed form of that anxiety varies over time. Isolated panic attacks are a short-term anxiety symptom that may appear with other disorders such as depression. Panic disorder is different, involving a disabling fear of experiencing future panic episodes.

Anxiety disorders commonly run in families; thus, when a child is given an anxiety disorder diagnosis, you may find that either or both parents likely have struggled with anxiety disorders themselves. This familial tendency can occur through shared genetic traits, through children absorbing the anxious sentiments a parent generates within the household, or both. In some situations, the most effective way to help an anxious child is to help the parent to manage the parent's own anxiety more effectively and thus create a more stable and supportive home environment for the child.

Strategies shown to be effective for treating anxiety in children include different forms of psychotherapy in which support for exposure to feared thoughts or ideas is their most common element (Chorpita and Daleiden 2009). Repeated exposure to feared situations or memories that do not have any negative consequences, through repetition and reframing, will help the child's mind unlearn that fear. However, if that fear is still a real one, such as when a traumatized child is still at risk for future abuse, then psychotherapy alone will not be as beneficial until the child's safety is secured. CBT is the most commonly available modality for anxiety treatment that uses exposure (Dickson et al. 2022).

Parents also must challenge or restrict the avoidance behaviors in their child because avoidance of a feared situation leads to a temporary relief of anxiety that over time reinforces the fear and worsens the severity of the anxiety. For instance, a fear of attending school becomes stronger if the child is allowed to repeatedly skip school. SSRIs, including sertraline and fluoxetine, have been shown in many studies to be effective in treating different forms of childhood anxiety disorders and are most effective when used in combination with psychotherapy (Mohatt et al. 2014).

OCD and PTSD are anxiety-related diagnoses that are listed in their own diagnostic classes of DSM-5-TR: "Obsessive-Compulsive and Related Disorders" (which includes hoarding disorder and trichotillomania) and "Trauma- and Stressor-Related Disorders" (which includes acute stress disorder and adjustment disorders), respectively. OCD responds very well to the same first-line therapies used for other anxiety disorders: CBT and SSRIs. PTSD has been found to respond well to exposure-based therapies such as trauma-focused CBT, but its response to medications in children is not so well established.

Recurrent or Excessive Physical Complaints

Primary care clinicians know that recurrent headaches, chest pain, nausea, and fatigue are the presenting concern in about 10% of all office visits by adolescents, and recurrent abdominal pain alone is the presenting concern in about 5% of all pediatric office visits (Silber 2011). Although these somatic complaints may have many etiologies, the most common etiologies are psychiatric. Knowing this, whenever we hear a psychosomatic complaint, we consider whether anxiety disorders, depressive disorders, or adjustment disorders are the cause. Treatments for anxiety and depression are both effective and straightforward. The treatments for somatic disorders (somatic symptom disorder, factitious disorder, conversion disorder) are more challenging, so we consider them after ruling out anxiety and depressive disorders (Table 4–7).

We do not, however, favor considering somatic disorders only after excluding all possible causes for somatic complaints. Contemporary medicine overvalues biological explanations for somatic symptoms and usually leaves other explanations, including psychiatric etiologies, as diagnoses of exclusion. The following are unfortunate effects of a medical-before-psychiatric approach:

- Mental illness may go unrecognized.
- Patients and parents may react poorly to hearing an "it is all in your head" sort of explanation after multiple investigations and appointments.
- Families may try to prove that symptoms are real and insist on inappropriate tests or procedures.
- Acceptance of psychiatric care or forms of appropriate functional assistance may be decreased.

To counteract these pitfalls, we recommend describing psychiatric etiologies to families when presenting your *initial* somatic symptom differential diagnosis and then openly discussing them throughout. You can do this by describing what you think are the most likely psychobiological pathways for somatic symptoms. For instance, you can explain how stress affects the autonomic nervous system, which can lower gastric pH and alter intestinal motility (for nausea and abdominal pain) or can alter blood vessel smooth muscle tone (for headaches). By offering a biological account for physical symptoms of a mental illness, you will help patients and their caregivers more readily accept psychiatric interventions such as CBT and relaxation therapy because you have taught them that psychiatric intervention can modify the functioning of the autonomic nervous system.

Children with somatic symptom disorders usually lack awareness that stress or anxiety is linked to their physical experiences or may lack an ability to adequately use words to describe their emotional states (referred to as *alexithymia*).

TABLE 4–7. Screening questions for recurrent or excessive physical complaints

Suggested questions

First consider

Abuse or maltreatment	*"Has anything or anyone made you feel uncomfortable or unsafe?"*
	(for caregiver) *"Has anything happened to your child that really shouldn't have happened?"*
Adjustment disorder	*"Did something stressful happen in the 3 months before these symptoms appeared?"*
Anxiety disorders	(for caregiver) *"Does your child have a lot of worries that cause distress?"*
Depressive disorders	(for caregiver) *"Has your child's mood been unusually down or low for more than a couple of weeks?"*

Common diagnostic possibilities

Conversion disorder	For clinician: consider when you identify a loss of motor or sensory function that is inconsistent with recognized disorders.
Factitious disorder imposed on self	(for caregiver—asked away from the child) *"Do you suspect your child may be intentionally exaggerating symptoms?"*
Factitious disorder imposed on another	For clinician: consider when the parent has a pattern of reporting symptoms in the child inconsistent with recognized disorders.
Panic attacks	*"Do you experience sudden surges of fear that make your body feel shaky or your heart race?"*
Somatic symptom disorder	(for caregiver) *"Does your child have recurrent physical symptoms that disrupt their daily life? Does your child have an excessive focus on their physical symptoms?"*

The classic childhood pattern is that somatic symptoms increase before stressful experiences, such as attending school, visiting someone else's home, or performing publicly, but decrease if stressful situations are avoided. Specifically experienced symptoms may change over time, in that a child with recurrent abdominal pain early in life may develop recurrent headaches and fatigue as a teenager.

In the case of a conversion disorder with prominent unusual motor problems (such as paralysis of only one shoulder) or sensory problems (such as a loss of all feeling in the legs with normal reflexes) that do not follow logical neurological patterns, we similarly find it important to help the child exit their presentation without accusing them of having biologically false symptoms. For instance, you can explain to a patient that your examination identified no major medical difficulties but that in your experience other young people with similar symptoms experienced a rapid resolution. A face-saving explanation such as *"I believe that in a short time your nerves will simply reset themselves, like how the seasons change"* may be particularly helpful. Successfully responding to conversion symptoms relies as much on the art of medicine as on the science of medicine.

A young person also may intentionally falsify symptoms to malinger when there is a clear secondary gain or as part of a factitious disorder. Detecting a case of factitious disorder imposed on another requires a clinician to mentally shift their thinking to consider this possibility because it is difficult to accept that a caregiver might misrepresent, simulate, or cause signs of illness in their child. Suspected cases of factitious disorder are best managed by all of a patient's clinicians communicating directly with one another about their concerns, consulting local experts on this topic, and then arriving at a unified rather than divided approach to helping the child.

Sleep Problems

Sleep problems are very common, present in 5%–20% of children (Meltzer et al. 2010) and even more common in children with underlying psychiatric and neurological disorders (DelRosso et al. 2021). Most childhood insomnia can be traced to poor sleep habits and inadequate enforcement of bedtime habits by caregivers. The contemporary incorporation of electronics into every aspect of daily life means that it is no longer sufficient for clinicians to simply recommend no television in the bedroom of a child with insomnia. Cell phones have become sleep prevention devices through the applications, text and instant messaging, and games they bring right into the child's bed. Restricting all computer access, video games, and cell phone use after a certain time in the evening can yield a dramatic improvement in the amount of sleep that children (and their caregivers) get.

Another key sleep hygiene problem is a loss of the behavioral association that being in bed equals sleep time. Behavioral routines around going to bed help signal to the brain when it is time to disconnect. Doing homework in bed, eating in bed, playing in bed, and communicating with friends from bed break that behavioral association. For those with insomnia, the act of lying awake in bed for a long time, staring at the clock, and waiting for sleep can become another sleep-interfering behavior. If sleep does not come quickly, the behavioral association that bed equals sleep is improved by getting out of the bed for a nonelectronic quiet activity such as sitting in a chair to read and returning to bed only when feeling sleepy. A list of sleep hygiene practices appears in Chapter 15, "Initiating Psychosocial Interventions."

Sleep is also impaired by distracting thoughts, worries, or symptoms of many different DSM-5-TR conditions (Table 4–8). Addressing problems such as maltreatment, PTSD, anxiety, and mood disorders can significantly improve sleep. In some cases, insomnia worsens or perpetuates a mood disorder to such a degree that using a medication to restore adequate sleep can be a way to help resolve that mood disorder more quickly.

Reasonable bedtimes may be a sticking point to address. Caregivers cannot expect adolescents to fall asleep at 8:00 P.M. every night, even though that may be a reasonable expectation for younger children. For children with long-term sleep phase advancement problems, such as rarely falling asleep before 3:00 A.M., changing bedtimes too quickly does not work because it takes weeks to retrain the circadian rhythm and behavioral associations with sleep.

Obstructive sleep apnea also can have negative psychiatric effects; thus, when apnea is found in a (typically obese) child through polysomnography, a sleep apnea treatment also may improve other psychiatric symptoms. When the tonsils are large, a tonsillectomy or adenoidectomy may be helpful. Any more extensive surgical intervention on the palate or pharynx of a growing child should be viewed with much greater skepticism because of higher rates of complications. Continuous positive airway pressure (CPAP) systems can be effective and safe for sleep apnea treatment, but it is

TABLE 4–8. Screening questions for sleep problems

	Suggested questions
First consider	
Abuse	*"Has anything or anyone made you feel uncomfortable or unsafe?"*
	(for caregiver) *"Has anything happened to your child that really shouldn't have happened?"*
Bullying	*"Have other kids been teasing you or making you feel afraid?"*
Poor sleep habits	*"What is your routine before going to bed? What do you do when you cannot sleep?"*
Common diagnostic possibilities	
Generalized anxiety disorder	*"Do you feel tense, restless, or worried most of the time? Do these worries keep you awake?"*
Insomnia disorder	*"Have you had difficulty with sleep 3 or more nights a week for at least the past 3 months?"*
Major depressive disorder	*"Have you felt really down, depressed, or uninterested in things you used to enjoy for more than 2 weeks?"*
PTSD	*"Do you avoid reminders of traumatic events in your past? Do you startle easily or get frequent nightmares?"*

typically difficult to get a child to use a CPAP machine every night—far more often, these systems are purchased but not used. Note that with severe sleep apnea, potent sedatives such as benzodiazepines at night are recommended.

Parents and patients often ask for a prescribed medication to help with sleep. The challenges of this strategy include limitations in effectiveness, a psychological association that one cannot sleep without a pill, physiological dependence or tolerance, and exposure to unwanted adverse effects. After sleep hygiene measures fail, we may consider using a medication to treat moderate to severe insomnia in children, but the core principle should be to favor nonaddictive, safe sedative options with few side effects. The secondary principle is that if a child has insomnia plus another psychiatric disorder, selecting a medication that can address both conditions at once is preferred to using multiple medications.

Antihistamines are a reasonable first-line option because of their safety profile. Melatonin, up to 5 mg nightly, is considered generally safe, but at least theoretical concerns exist about the negative effects it may have on other hormone systems. More potent sedative options include the α_2-agonists (clonidine, guanfacine), which, when administered nightly, could help with sleep in addition to other conditions such as ADHD. Anxiety that continues to cause insomnia despite the use of SSRIs and CBT may benefit from hydroxyzine as a nonaddictive option or an off-label trial of a sedating antidepressant such as mirtazapine. In very severe cases, a low dose of a benzodiazepine or an off-label benzodiazepine analogue (zolpidem, zaleplon) might be necessary to achieve results. For children requiring an antipsychotic to treat their psychiatric disorder, a sedating option such as quetiapine or risperidone taken at bedtime may improve the comorbid insomnia. Use of an antipsychotic solely as a sleep aid is inappropriate and not recommended for children (McVoy and Findling 2013).

Self-Harm and Suicidality

Suicidality and self-harm behaviors are very common among adolescents, more common than many people realize. In a national survey, 18.8% of high school students self-reported seriously considering suicide, and 8.9% reported having attempted suicide in the previous year (Ivey-Stephenson et al. 2020). Thankfully, completed suicides are far rarer than suicide attempts. You are more likely to get full and honest answers about suicidality and substance abuse when interviewing a young person away from their caregivers, so ask for privacy before you ask about self-harm (Table 4–9).

Asking young people whether they feel suicidal can be awkward until you become accustomed to doing it. Despite the awkward feelings, these questions cannot be avoided. Because suicide is one of the three leading causes of death among young people, asking a young person about feelings of suicide is just as important as screening an adult for chest pain or shortness of breath.

If you fear that asking about suicide creates risks, allow us to put your mind at ease. Asking about suicidal thoughts, plans, and past actions not only enables you to gather essen-

TABLE 4–9. Screening questions for self-harm and suicidality

	Suggested questions
First consider	
Risk acuity[a]	*"Have you ever thought about hurting yourself or taking your own life? Have you ever done something to hurt yourself or tried to kill yourself? Do you have any plans now for how you would kill yourself?"*
Current triggers[a]	*"Do you have any recent relationship problems or big disappointments?"*
Current supports[a]	*"Do you have anyone in your life who helps support you?"*
Access to lethal means[a]	*"Can you easily get a gun or enough pills that you think could kill you?"*
Common diagnostic possibilities	
Bipolar disorder	*"Has there ever been a period of a week or more when you were the opposite of depressed, with super high energy and little need for sleep?"*
Major depressive disorder	*"Have you felt really down, depressed, or uninterested in things you used to enjoy for more than 2 weeks?"*
Persistent depressive disorder	*"Have you felt persistently sad or gloomy for more than a year?"*
Substance use disorder[a]	*"Have you been using drugs or alcohol?"*

[a]These questions should be asked when the patient is alone.

tial diagnostic information but also shows your concern. For a self-harming or suicidal young person, having an adult in their life who communicates that they care about them is therapeutic.

When asking about suicidality, we suggest starting with broad questions, then getting specific. Asking *"Have you ever…?"* risk questions before *"How about now…?"* questions just flows better conversationally. If you uncover self-harm or suicidal behaviors, continuing to ask questions about previous suicidal behaviors (the strongest predictor of future behavior), current plans to self-harm, and current stressors is key to being able to understand the immediacy of any risks. If you learn that the adolescent tried to avoid premature discovery of a suicide attempt, such as by hiding empty pill bottles, this would be very concerning. Easy, impulsive access to lethal means, such as a loaded firearm, is another major risk factor.

Recurrent self-harm behaviors, such as cutting, are often cited by young people themselves as a coping mechanism that they perform in part to reduce their risk of suicide. However, recurrent self-harm increases the risk for future suicidal behaviors.

The strongest predictors of a future suicide are a history of suicide attempts, an active mood disorder, current substance abuse, and a family history of suicidal behavior. For adolescents in particular, suicide attempts are often triggered after an acute loss or disappointment, such as a breakup with a boyfriend or girlfriend or an acute family conflict. Nearly 90% of adolescent suicide deaths occur from firearms or suffocation, which includes hanging, so suicidal plans involving these strategies are the most concerning (Eaton et al. 2008). Suicide attempts by overdose are much more common but are also much less likely to be lethal.

We suggest that after learning both the general and the specific details of the situation, you keep in mind a prudent layperson standard for when to consider an acute hospitalization. Child mental health specialists are not much better than anyone else would be at assessing risks once all the details of a situation are known. The difference is that child mental health specialists excel at eliciting the details of a situation. The key is to keep asking for more information to flesh out the whole situation rather than stopping your inquiries at "they said they feel suicidal." You should consider hospitalization for any young person who appears to have a significant safety risk after you elicit the details of the situation. Psychiatric hospitalization keeps a patient physically safe for at least a short time while further steps in their care can be initiated.

Young people with recurrent self-harm behavior or significant suicidal thoughts should be referred for psychotherapy because this is clearly the most effective treatment available. If a family declines to use counseling with a mental health professional, you can also encourage the use of as many other social supports and supervision arrangements as possible.

Medications do not have a significant role in reducing suicide or self-harm risks on a short-term basis. However, if a child has major depressive disorder or an anxiety disorder, then long-term suicide risks can be reduced through successful treatment with SSRIs. See Chapter 16, "Starting a Psychotherapy," for more information about SSRI use and suicidality. For a severe depression, the greatest treatment responses occur when SSRIs are combined with psychotherapy. Frequent monitoring and making the environment safe (e.g., restricting access to dangerous medications and firearms) are advised for all suicidal young people.

Substance Abuse

The key to making any diagnosis is thinking of the possibility, which can be a challenge when it comes to adolescent substance abuse (Table 4–10). When we see fresh-faced, youthful adolescents in our offices, we can find it hard to simultaneously view them as possible substance abusers. The available statistics dictate that we do so. In the United States alone, national surveys show that 7% of 12- to 17-year-olds used alcohol in the past month, and 6.7% used nicotine vape or tobacco. Moreover, 10.5% of 12- to 17-year-olds used marijuana in the past year, 3.3% misused prescription medications (stimulants, benzodiazepines, narcotics), 2.4% used inhalants, 1.3% used hallucinogens (LSD, mushrooms), and 0.7% abused dextromethorphan (Substance Abuse and Mental Health Services Administration 2022).

Recognition starts with remembering to ask about substance use and ideally doing so without a parent in the room. We prefer to ask parents to leave the room for this aspect of the encounter and openly reemphasize applicable confidentiality rules during the separation process. In general, everyone understands the concept of maintaining confidentiality unless a major safety risk exists, such as having blackouts or driving while intoxicated. This same one-on-one time can be used to discuss other sensitive topics such as self-harm and suicidality.

A widely recommended screening tool for adolescents is the CRAFFT (Car, Relax, Alone, Forget, Friends, Trouble; Figure 4–1), which the American Academy of Pediatrics recom-

TABLE 4–10. Screening questions for substance abuse

	Suggested questions
First consider	
Safety[a]	*"Have you ever been in a car driven by someone who was drunk or high? Have you injured yourself while you were drunk or high? Have you blacked out or done things you regret while drunk or high?"*
Common diagnostic possibilities	
Substance use disorder[a]	*"Have people asked you to cut down on drinking or using drugs? Do you ever drink or use drugs when you are alone? Do you get strong cravings or end up using more than you wanted to?"*
Substance withdrawal	*"Do you get more moody or anxious while your alcohol or drugs are wearing off?"*
Substance tolerance	*"Has the same amount of drug or alcohol been losing its effect over time?"*
Substance/ medication-induced mental disorder	*"Did you develop more mood or anxiety problems after you started using?"*
Self-medication role of substances	*"Are there any problems that you wanted the alcohol or drugs to resolve?"*

[a]These questions should be asked when the patient is alone.

mends using during adolescent health maintenance appointments (Yuma Guerrero et al. 2012). If two or more answers are positive, there is a high chance of a substance use disorder being present (Knight et al. 2002).

Urine drug testing may help you evaluate the cause of an acute intoxication or may be used for tracking care within a specialized substance abuse treatment program. However, we do not otherwise recommend urine drug testing as a part of routine care because it can unnecessarily diminish the therapeutic alliance.

Begin: *"I'm going to ask you a few questions that I ask all my patients. Please be honest. I will keep your answers confidential."*

Part A
During the PAST 12 MONTHS, on how many days did you:

1. Drink more than a few sips of beer, wine, or any drink containing **alcohol**? Say "0" if none.   `___ # of days`

2. Use any **marijuana** (cannabis, weed, oil, wax, or hash by smoking, vaping, dabbing, or in edibles) or **synthetic marijuana** (like "K2," "Spice")? Say "0" if none.   `___ # of days`

3. Use **anything else to get high** (like other illegal drugs, pills, prescription or over-the-counter medications, and things that you sniff, huff, vape, or inject)? Say "0" if none.   `___ # of days`

Did the patient answer "0" for all questions in Part A?

Yes ☐   No ☐

↓   ↓

Ask 1ˢᵗ question only in Part B, then STOP   **Ask all 6 questions in Part B**

Part B		Circle one
C	Have you ever ridden in a **CAR** driven by someone (including yourself) who was "high" or had been using alcohol or drugs?	No Yes
R	Do you ever use alcohol or drugs to **RELAX**, feel better about yourself, or fit in?	No Yes
A	Do you ever use alcohol or drugs while you are by yourself, or **ALONE**?	No Yes
F	Do you ever **FORGET** things you did while using alcohol or drugs?	No Yes
F	Do your **FAMILY** or **FRIENDS** ever tell you that you should cut down on your drinking or drug use?	No Yes
T	Have you ever gotten into **TROUBLE** while you were using alcohol or drugs?	No Yes

***Two or more YES answers in Part B suggests a serious problem that needs further assessment. See back for further instructions** ⟶

FIGURE 4–1.   The CRAFFT Screening Interview.

©John R. Knight, MD, Boston Children's Hospital, 2022. Reproduced with permission from the Center for Adolescent Behavioral Health Research (CABHRe), Boston Children's Hospital. For more information and versions in other languages, see www.crafft.org.

In the past, the emphasis was on needing to determine whether a patient's substance use represented abuse or dependence. Because this differentiation was often unclear and carried both stigma and legal ramifications, these separate dependence and abuse diagnoses were merged into a single substance use disorder diagnosis in DSM-5. The hallmarks of a substance use disorder include loss of control over one's use, social impairments, use in risky situations or despite negative consequences, and physiological changes due to tolerance or withdrawal. In other words, not all adolescents who use substances have a disorder.

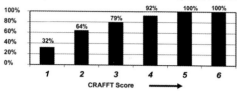

CRAFFT Score Interpretation

Probability of a DSM-5 Substance Use Disorder by CRAFFT score*

*Data source: Mitchell SG, Kelly SM, Gryczynski J, Myers CP, O'Grady KE, Kirk AS, & Schwartz RP. (2014). The CRAFFT cut-points and DSM-5 criteria for alcohol and other drugs: a reevaluation and reexamination. Substance Abuse, 35(4), 376–80.

- -

Use the 5 R's talking points for brief counseling.

1. **REVIEW** screening results
   For each "yes" response: *"Can you tell me more about that?"*

2. **RECOMMEND** not to use
   "As your doctor (nurse/health care provider), my recommendation is not to use any alcohol, marijuana or other drug because they can: 1) Harm your developing brain; 2) Interfere with learning and memory, and 3) Put you in embarrassing or dangerous situations."

3. **RIDING/DRIVING** risk counseling
   "Motor vehicle crashes are the leading cause of death for young people. I give all my patients the Contract for Life. Please take it home and discuss it with your parents/guardians to create a plan for safe rides home."

4. **RESPONSE** elicit self-motivational statements
   Non-users: *"If someone asked you why you don't drink or use drugs, what would you say?"* Users: *"What would be some of the benefits of not using?"*

5. **REINFORCE** self-efficacy
   "I believe you have what it takes to keep alcohol and drugs from getting in the way of achieving your goals."

Give patient Contract for Life. Available at www.crafft.org/contract

FIGURE 4–1.   The CRAFFT Screening Interview. *(continued)*
©John R. Knight, MD, Boston Children's Hospital, 2022. Reproduced with permission from the Center for Adolescent Behavioral Health Research (CABHRe), Boston Children's Hospital. For more information and versions in other languages, see www.crafft.org.

Be alert to symptoms caused by substance abuse that resemble another psychiatric illness. Sedative drugs (hypnotics, anxiolytics, and alcohol) can cause depression during intoxication but anxiety during withdrawal. Stimulating drugs (amphetamines, cocaine) can cause psychosis and anxiety during intoxication but depression during withdrawal. Both drug classes cause sexual and sleep disturbances. Psychotic symptoms may occur from anticholinergics, cardiovascular drugs, steroids, stimulants, and depressants. Marijuana can cause depressed mood and anxiety, even though adolescents claim that it treats their depression or anxiety. In an adolescent vulnerable to psychosis, marijuana can trigger persisting psychotic symptoms (Morin et al. 2019; van Nierop et al. 2013).

When substance-created psychiatric symptoms are possible, we motivate the adolescent to do a self-test of not using for a specific period (e.g., at least 2 weeks) to see what happens. Most substance-induced mental disorders will begin improving after a few weeks of abstinence after the person gets through a spike in cravings. For adolescents who say "I can stop whenever I want to," we would follow this statement by empowering them to do just that for whatever reasons that make the most sense to them—with reasons to quit ideally identified through a motivational interviewing process. This does two things: 1) it determines whether their symptoms really are substance induced; and 2) if they cannot go more than 2 weeks without using, it highlights for them their lack of control over their use.

Care for a substance use disorder is based on educating adolescents about the negative outcomes of use, helping them learn their triggers and motivating reasons to use, building motivation for change, and shaping family involvement in resolving the problem. Motivational interviewing, CBT, family therapy, supervised peer groups, mindfulness training, identifying triggers (to avoid future cue-based use), changing peer groups, and arranging for rewards for evidence of sobriety are all specific outpatient care options.

Disturbed Eating

Eating disorders such as anorexia and bulimia can present a diagnostic challenge in that young people who have become significantly ill with an eating disorder generally try to hide their symptoms, even when asked directly by a trusted person (Table 4–11). With low-weight anorexia nervosa, withholding information or even lying to clinicians often happens in the service of maintaining disordered eating. Therapists sometimes refer to these lies as the eating disorder, rather than the patient themselves, doing the talking. Because of this inconsistency, collateral informants (i.e., parents and other caregivers) are typically very helpful for understanding the extent of symptoms and behaviors. Taking an investiga-

TABLE 4–11. Screening questions for disturbed eating

	Suggested questions
First consider	
Medically induced weight loss	*"Have you had recurring diarrhea?"* (inflammatory bowel disease) *"Have you been losing weight despite wanting to maintain?"* (endocrine disorder or malignancy)
Self-harm[a]	"Have you been thinking about hurting yourself? Have you ever hurt yourself or attempted suicide?"
Common diagnostic possibilities	
Anorexia nervosa	*"Do you worry about losing control when you eat? Do you prefer to eat alone?"* (growth curve: an unexpected weight loss or failure to gain appropriately)
Bulimia nervosa	*"Have you had recurring times when you overeat and then feel the need to compensate afterward? Do you use laxatives or vomit after meals?"*
Major depressive disorder	*"Have you felt really down, depressed, or uninterested in things you used to enjoy for more than 2 weeks?"*
Substance use disorder[a]	*"Have you been using drugs or alcohol?"*

[a]These questions should be asked when the patient is alone.

tive approach helps. When you learn that a young person who denies self-induced vomiting goes to the bathroom immediately after most of their meals, you should explore the possibility of disturbed eating and body image. Remember that young people with eating disorders often show rigid thinking and perfectionism.

Postpartum Maternal Mental Health

Maternal peripartum depression is common, with frequencies reported as higher in developing countries (about 1 in 5) than in developed countries (about 1 in 10) (Paschetta et al. 2014). The risk that the mother of a newborn will experience depression increases with stressors such as poverty, lack of partner support, unwanted pregnancy, and domestic violence. When a woman has depressive symptoms during her pregnancy, the chances that she will develop postpartum depression increase, so we counsel increased vigilance for these parents.

Postdelivery obstetric care for mothers and the first year of health maintenance care for children ideally include some form of screening for maternal problems with depression and anxiety (Table 4–12). You can accomplish this by conversationally asking the mother about her psychological well-being (which helps to communicate its importance) and can supplement this approach with a brief rating scale screen (such as the 9-item Patient Health Questionnaire, Edinburgh Postnatal Depression Scale, or 7-item Generalized Anxiety Disorder scale) in routine office care. Fatigue and poor sleep, which are often associated with parenthood itself, need to be recognized as potential signs of an episode of major depressive disorder.

Good parental mental health is important for children. When parents struggle, this can have negative effects on the child's physical state (poor health, poor weight gain), cognitive status (delayed acquisition of milestones, impaired attention), social development (oppositional defiant disorder, conduct problems), behavior (more crying, irritability, and temperament challenges), or emotional development (depression, anxiety) (Satyanarayana et al. 2011). In rare instances, a parental mental health condition, such as a developing psychosis, can become so severe that the parent will harm the child.

Treating parental mental health problems during a child's early development positively affects a child's mental health. When a parent or other caregiver with mental illness receives care, this also greatly increases the chance that the child will develop an easygoing temperament, which will pay dividends in the household for years (Hanington et al. 2010).

Treating a parent or caregiver begins with addressing life stressors ranging from mild (keeping up with laundry or cleaning) to severe (loss of employment, poor relationship with a partner). Rallying a parent's personal care system to support them and take their distress seriously may be sufficient to produce positive change. Psychotherapy is indicated

TABLE 4–12. Screening questions for postpartum maternal mental health

	Suggested questions
First consider	
Suicidality	*"Have you been having thoughts about hurting yourself?"*
Psychosis	*"Have you been hearing voices or feeling worried that your mind is playing tricks on you?"*
Child safety	*"Have you felt worried that you might intentionally hurt your child?"*
Common diagnostic possibilities	
Anxiety disorder	*"Do you feel tense or worried most of the time? Do worries affect your sleep?"*
Major depressive disorder	*"Have you felt really down, depressed, or uninterested in things you used to enjoy for more than 2 weeks?"*

for any situations in which major depression, generalized anxiety disorder, or another significant disorder has set in.

When deciding whether to use psychiatric medications postpartum, keep in mind the same things you would consider for mental health treatment at any other time. The amount of psychiatric medication transmitted through breast milk is typically too low to have any effects on a breastfeeding child, with the notable exception of lithium (Davanzo et al. 2011). Moderate to severe depression generally responds most quickly to a combination of SSRIs and psychotherapy, so this should be the usual approach (Lanza di Scalea and Wisner 2009). Brexanolone, the first FDA-approved medication for the treatment of postpartum depression, is a manufactured version of allopregnanolone, a molecule the body usually makes from progesterone. Brexanolone is an intravenous infusion administered in a hospital treatment center over 2.5 days. The use of brexanolone is clinically limited because of the difficulty of administering it and its current cost (Meltzer-Brody et al. 2018).

Medication choices during pregnancy itself must be weighed a bit more carefully against the potential effects a specific medication may have on a developing fetus. The traditional advice was to avoid lithium because of the risk of Eb-stein anomaly, but more recent research (Pearlstein 2013) identifies those congenital defects of the tricuspid valve as rarer than previously believed. Lithium may be prescribed, with caution and counseling, during pregnancy (Fornaro et al. 2020). We do, however, advise against the use of valproate, a known teratogen whose use by mothers is associated with neurodevelopmental disorders in children. The rare, but well-reported, risk of low birth weight or pulmonary hypertension in the newborn from SSRI use during pregnancy means that SSRIs should be reserved for more severe cases of depression and anxiety (Pearlstein 2013). Any time a parent develops psychosis or suicidality, a hospital admission level of care should be considered.

Chapter 5

Reaching a DSM-5-TR Diagnosis When You Have 15 Minutes

Even the most seasoned and skilled practitioner would like at least 30 minutes to perform a diagnostic mental health interview. Determining the character traits, cognitive ability, and emotional health of another person, especially a child or an adolescent, is difficult. So why even discuss a 15-minute diagnostic interview as a basis for reaching any DSM-5-TR diagnoses?

Short diagnostic mental health interviews are certainly not ideal, but they are the daily reality faced by many of those who care for young people. Primary care and emergency department clinicians are routinely expected to perform brief, efficient interviews. Pediatric primary care clinicians can be expected to evaluate as many as 30 different children per day, which leaves only about 15 minutes to spend with each patient. Emergency department clinicians are pressured to rapidly assess mental health concerns, particularly during evening hours when emergency environments are most stressed.

The time available for performing a mental health evaluation is further constrained when a patient or family fixates on physical health concerns instead. By the time you identify a psychiatric issue—the anxiety that precedes abdominal pain or the dysphoria experienced as a headache—you may have only a few minutes remaining in an appointment to conduct a full mental health diagnostic assessment. So it can help to begin encounters with physical chief complaints by setting expectations that you will address physical and mental health, by saying something like, *"Being healthy means caring for your mind, and your body, so I will ask about each."* It also helps to explain how much time you will have together. Patients often have the "Oh, by the way…" moments, when major mental health questions are broached seemingly as a clinician places their hand on the door to leave the examination room, so it helps to frame the encounter by offering something like, *"We will have 15 minutes together. Can we make sure to discuss both your mind and body needs in that time?"*

Clinicians frequently find their available time restricted in one way or another, so it helps to think about how to best use even a small amount of time to advance the care of children and adolescents with mental distress. The following five steps are one way to efficiently perform a focused mental health diagnostic assessment with a child or an adolescent:

1. Prescreen mental health concerns with a validated tool.
2. Identify the leading concerns.
3. Identify and address safety issues.
4. Diagnose a probable or unspecified disorder.
5. Recommend a next step.

Step 1: Use a Validated Tool to Prescreen Mental Health Concerns

While we always recommend the use of pre-interview assessment tools for well-child healthcare visits, we find them especially helpful when the chief complaint is a mental or behavioral health problem. Preassessment screening tools engage a patient and their caregivers in the treatment, normalize conversations about mental distress, and assist you in identifying the chief complaint. Several brief screening instruments for a wide variety of mental health concerns are available. One example is the DSM-5-TR (American Psychiatric Association 2022) Level 1 Cross-Cutting Symptom Measure, which lists selected symptoms of major DSM-5 disorders in a brief format. Versions exist for caregivers of children and adolescents between ages 6 and 17 and for patients between ages 11 and 17. These measures are free and can be reproduced for clinical use and are referenced further in Chapter 11, "Using DSM-5-TR Assessment Measures to Aid Diagnosis." We also recommend considering use of the Pediatric Symptom Checklist or the Strengths and Difficulties Questionnaire, two other brief but broad-based assessment measures that have the additional benefit of score validation for children in primary care medical settings.

Whatever screening tool you select for your practice setting, you should familiarize yourself with its scoring system. Most screening tools are designed to have high sensitivity, meaning that they aim to identify anyone who may have a particular diagnosis, but lower specificity, meaning that they will identify some persons for additional concern who ultimately will not have the diagnosis for which you are screening. Positive results in certain categories may suggest follow-up measures to use, such as a high inattention score on the DSM-5-TR Level 1 assessment being followed up with the DSM-5-TR Level 2 Inattention rating scale. Using follow-up measures can increase the efficiency of clinical encounters and, if patients are followed up over time, can be a good introduction to using validated scales to measure treatment response, relapse, and recovery. At the very least, the results of screening measures also can be used as conversation starters: *"I see that you indicated a few concerns in the questionnaire; can you tell me more about that?"*

Although the use of brief, broad screening measures is likely best for a fast-paced care facility, if time and the practice plan allow, a more detailed symptom checklist can be considered instead. These longer checklists will yield both information about many different individual areas of clinical functioning as compared against age-based norms, as well as predictions of the likelihood of specific clinical disorders being present. Two commonly utilized examples of such scales are the CBCL, Child Behavior Checklist (Achenbach 1991, 1992), and the BASC-3, Behavior Assessment System for Children, (Reynolds and Kamphaus 2015). While these tools take significantly more time for caregivers to complete and for office staff to score and interpret, they result in reliable, broad-based pictures of a young person's difficulties.

If you fail to recognize the presence of a mental health concern in advance, you can still pause an evaluation process when such concerns arise and ask for the symptom-focused screening information to be completed before continuing. For instance, you may say, "Given the concerns you just raised, could you take a few moments to complete this information, and I'll be back to discuss this more with you?" Taking this approach could allow you to proceed with seeing your next scheduled patient during that time and even have the assessment tool scored by an assistant while staying on schedule.

When you have identified a specific mental health concern, a condition- or symptom-focused rating scale could be used instead to provide better diagnostic information. Examples of focused DSM-5-TR scales include the Level 2 Cross-Cutting Symptom Measures for parents or children to characterize symptom categories such as anger, anxiety, depression, inattention, irritability, mania, sleep disturbance, somatic symptoms, and substance use; these scales are discussed in Chapter 11 but are also available online (www.psychiatry.org/Psychiatrists/Practice/DSM/Educational-Resources/DSM-5-Assessment-Measures). Other symptom-focused scales have been validated and normed with diagnostic score cutoffs in children and are discussed in Chapter 12, "Using Rating Scales and Alternative Diagnostic Systems While Assessing a Young Person." Positive results on these instruments more strongly suggest that a particular diagnosis is present, but the use of a diagnostic instrument ultimately relies on the prudent judgment of a practitioner.

Even the best rating scales and symptom checklists are inherently imperfect, so it is important to understand their limitations. Questions may be misunderstood, may miss key symptoms, may be influenced by a young person's or caregiver's tendency to overreport or underreport symptoms, or may be intentionally answered untruthfully. This is why all surveys and questionnaires must be followed up with a personalized diagnostic interview to yield a more reliable portrait. For instance, if you see an adolescent who denies having depression symptoms on their rating scale yet appears withdrawn, speaks in a low monotone, and describes feeling hopeless, depression must be considered, regardless of the scores on a symptom checklist.

Step 2: Identify the Leading Concerns

Once a pertinent rating scale has been completed and scored, the next step in a brief interview is to identify the young person's and caregiver's leading concern for further investigation. Identifying the leading concern can be as simple as asking specifically, "What are you most concerned about today?"

An unlimited list of concerns or complaints is too challenging to manage within a brief investigation, even if the concerns ultimately relate to the same diagnosis, as is often the case with depression. For instance, a family may describe sleep problems, poor academic performance, self-harm behavior, irritability, and conflict with a sibling as separate concerns. If you identify one of these areas, such as self-harm, as the chief concern for that day, with the understanding that remaining concerns such as sibling conflict may need to be addressed at another appointment, then a 15-minute interview can be more fruitful.

Your own careful judgment is the key. For example, if a patient and their caregivers are most concerned about sleep disturbances but your screening tools or examination alert you to a safety issue, you must explain to the caregivers that sleep disturbances are important, but the patient's safety is the leading concern.

Having the patient and their caregivers each identify a leading concern builds your therapeutic alliance and increases investment in your assessment and treatment. When a patient and his caregivers believe that you truly understand the leading concern, they are more likely to engage in treatment and follow the next steps you recommend.

Step 3: Identify and Address Safety Issues

Any mental health evaluation, no matter how brief, includes an assessment of safety. If you identify safety concerns, then the near-term care plan needs to account for how to reduce or eliminate that risk.

- If you suspect that self-harm or suicidal behaviors may occur, as when evaluating for depression, ask: "*Do you ever think about hurting yourself? Have you ever deliberately hurt yourself?*"
- If it is possible that abuse or neglect may be related to the reported symptoms, ask: "*Has anything made you feel uncomfortable or unsafe? Has anyone ever tried to hurt you?*"
- If it is possible that the child poses a risk to another person, ask: "*Have you ever hurt someone else on purpose? Do you have any plans to do that now?*"

Step 4: Diagnose a Probable or Unspecified Disorder

By inquiring about the circumstances and details surrounding a patient's (and their caregiver's) chief concern and reviewing the results of assessment tools, a practitioner can usually arrive at a probable diagnosis in 15 minutes. Confirmation of all but the most obvious diagnoses will take more assessment time or a future appointment to clarify. For instance, you might determine in just 15 minutes that a child has significant developmental impairments, leading to a diagnosis of unspecified neurodevelopmental disorder. Then, during their next appointment you would make more detailed inquiries to refine the diagnosis further, changing that diagnosis to something more specific such as a language disorder or an autism spectrum disorder.

In Chapter 4, "Working Together on Common Clinical Concerns," we outline the more likely diagnoses to consider and some specific screening questions you can use when confronted with common pediatric concerns.

Rapid assessments proceed more fruitfully with awareness of the key aspects of common clinical conditions. This is no different from the rest of medicine, in which shorthand understandings of disorders are used to guide clinical suspicion. When an adult reports chest pain radiating down his left arm, we suspect a heart attack. When a febrile infant pulls at their ears and acts grumpy, we suspect an ear infection. In a similar way, we can learn to recognize basic patterns of mental health. When a child experiences several weeks of a persistently low mood and loses interest in the activities and friends he usually enjoys, we suspect major depressive disorder. To help inform your clinical suspicion, Table 5–1 contains a list of common psychiatric conditions and shorthand descriptions. Additional information is available in later chapters.

Remember that these are descriptions of behaviors and symptoms. In isolation, these behaviors are not a diagnosis. In the DSM-5-TR system, for any constellation of behaviors and symptoms to qualify as a psychiatric diagnosis, they must meet two conditions:

1. They cause a significant functional impairment.
2. They are not better explained by another etiology.

The second rule is very important. A child can be inattentive for any number of reasons without having attention-deficit/hyperactivity disorder, and an adolescent can be sad for many reasons without experiencing a major depressive episode. If these kinds of behaviors and symptoms do not significantly impair function or can be better explained by another etiology, a formal mental health diagnosis should not be made.

TABLE 5–1. Shorthand descriptions of common DSM-5-TR diagnoses in children

Diagnosis	Description
Anorexia nervosa	Restrictive eating and food avoidance, often with an accompanying desire to avoid obesity, which persists despite negative consequences
Attention-deficit/ hyperactivity disorder	Developmentally inappropriate and persistent difficulty with inattention and/or hyperactivity with symptoms present in multiple settings
Autism spectrum disorder	A developmentally inappropriate and persistent pattern of predominant impairments in social relatedness and restricted interests and behaviors
Bipolar disorder	Discrete episode of elevated mood for multiple days with rapid thoughts, decreased need for sleep, persisting high energy, and unusual risk taking
Bulimia nervosa	More than 3 months of recurring episodes of binge eating followed by an intense desire to compensate afterward (e.g., by purging or using laxatives)
Conduct disorder	Repetitive significant violations of social rules and the rights of others over the course of a year
Encopresis	Inappropriate stool leakage with psychological adaptations, usually facilitated by chronic constipation
Generalized anxiety disorder	More than 6 months of persisting but diffuse, changing worries for more days than not that cause symptoms such as tension, fatigue, irritability, and poor concentration
Major depressive disorder	More than 2 weeks of low (or irritable) mood coupled with new neurovegetative symptoms (e.g., loss of concentration, low energy, altered sleep or appetite)

TABLE 5–1. Shorthand descriptions of common DSM-5-TR diagnoses in children *(continued)*

Diagnosis	Description
Obsessive-compulsive disorder	Time-consuming internal repetition of unwanted thoughts and/or a persistent focus on repeating specific types of behaviors or mental acts (e.g., cleaning, counting)
Oppositional defiant disorder	Developmentally inappropriate opposition to and defiance of adult rules and requests for more than 6 months
Panic attack	Sudden worry or fear accompanied by body symptoms such as a racing heart rate and physiological arousal (panic disorder considered if recurring attacks are feared and are affecting function)
Phobia (social or specific)	Excessive fear of an object or a situation that causes a dysfunctional degree of avoidance and distress for > 6 months
Posttraumatic stress disorder	A traumatic experience has led to avoidance of trauma reminders, hypervigilance to future threats, and unwanted reexperiencing (including nightmares) for > 1 month

Source. American Psychiatric Association 2022.

Alternately, clinicians may make an *unspecified* diagnosis when a young person experiences symptoms characteristic of a mental disorder that cause clinically significant distress but do not meet the full criteria for a named diagnosis. If a clinician wishes to communicate the specific reason that symptoms in a child or an adolescent do not meet criteria, the practitioner is encouraged to use the *other specified* diagnosis. In a 15-minute diagnostic interview, clinicians may be more likely to arrive at unspecified diagnostic labels rather than full diagnoses, but this should be a reminder of the need for additional diagnostic clarification later.

You can (and should) plan to follow up with the child or adolescent to see how these symptoms either resolve or develop into a specific diagnosis. Children and adolescents deserve the most accurate and specific diagnosis possible.

Step 5: Recommend a Next Step

Treat versus refer decisions end up being based on patient factors, such as diagnosis and severity, along with the fit between a patient's treatment needs and your abilities and availabilities as a clinician and the type of services available in your local community.

Therapist Referral

For nearly every moderate or severe mental health problem, referring a child or an adolescent to a skilled mental health therapist is essential. Explaining why you think seeing a therapist will be helpful may increase motivation for patients and caregivers to follow through on your referral. If caregivers have reservations about working with a mental health clinician, it helps to address those concerns during the referral and to normalize the referral by saying something like *"Just as I would refer you to a specialist to examine your eyes if I thought you needed glasses, I recommend that you see a mental health specialist for the concerns we have identified together."*

Family and Self-Care-Delivered Interventions

For low-severity problems, it may be appropriate to provide coaching on behavior or life management changes a patient and his caregivers can make at home. Providing guidance on how to improve sleep hygiene, to manage a problem behavior, or to support a young person through a life adjustment is an everyday occurrence for most primary care clinicians, and we provide some guidance in Chapter 15, "Psychosocial Interventions." Handout instructions, books, videos, or Web sites so that the family can obtain additional guidance after the appointment also may be of assistance.

Educational Assessment

For children struggling in school for whom a learning disability is a consideration, we advocate for educational testing. The route for doing this may hinge on motivating the parent to make a written request for a learning disability assessment at the child's school, which is required in some settings, including the United States.

Early Intervention Services Referral

For very young children with developmental concerns, refer the child to a local early intervention program. In the United States, this involves the federally sponsored Zero to Three program (www.zerotothree.org) or a school district–sponsored program for children ages 4–5 years.

Safety Plan

For a significant suicide, homicide, or other behavior-related safety risk, an immediate safety plan or hospitalization should be explored with the local mental health crisis system. For milder risks such as depression without active suicidal thoughts or plans, appropriate parental supervision and monitoring would be enough to detect any worsening risks.

Medications

It is usually inappropriate to recommend a new long-term psychotropic medication after only a 15-minute assessment. The exception might be a short-term trial of an over-the-counter medication with low medical side-effect risks, such as melatonin to help with insomnia. However, after a second appointment or any evaluation of a longer duration when the diagnosis becomes more certain, a prescription may be appropriate. Whenever you suspect more severe mental disorders, such as bipolar disorder or schizophrenia, you should refer a patient and their caregivers immediately to a specialty mental health practitioner.

Follow-Up Appointment

If you identify a mental disorder, recommend a follow-up appointment. This can serve several purposes:

- Provide enough time to better complete the diagnostic process
- Communicate your ongoing therapeutic connection and support around the problem

- Track the response to any initial intervention so that the treatment plan can be adjusted
- Identify any problems with the referral plan, creating an opportunity for resolution

Chapter 6

Reaching a DSM-5-TR Diagnosis When You Have 30 Minutes

In Chapter 5, "Reaching a DSM-5-TR Diagnosis When You Have 15 Minutes," we described an approach to the diagnostic process to take when your time with a patient is limited to 15 minutes. Now we loosen things up a bit and discuss a more overall diagnostically reasonable scenario in which you have more time available to spend with your patient—around half an hour. We do not recommend conducting interview and diagnostic processes under arbitrarily imposed time restrictions, but we want to reflect the realities of clinical practice: scheduling restrictions do exist, and even without a forced time crunch, there is value in organizing one's diagnostic process to be most efficient.

Every interview with a young person with mental distress will be unique. Sometimes you will need to calm a screaming child or warm up a reluctant adolescent before you can ask any diagnostic questions. In moments like these, it sometimes feels like you are wasting time. You have other people to see and other tasks to attend to. However, good interviewers learn to receive these moments as part of the interview itself. They watch and listen to the child or adolescent for clues about whether the distress is internal or external and what events bring them into and out of engagement with a practitioner.

Every young person is also unique, so we begin an initial encounter by getting to know the child or adolescent we are seeing. We use different strategies depending on the child's age and developmental status, the location in which we are meeting, our familiarity with the patient, the patient's sense of humor, and many other variables. Before introducing ourselves to a patient, we like to know how long they have been waiting and with whom. A child who has sat calmly for 15 minutes in a waiting room will likely have different needs from the same child who has been waiting hours to see you in the emergency department. When we meet a patient, we prefer to open the conversation with a topic in which the child or adolescent is already engaged. If a young child brings a stuffed animal to an appointment or wears a colorful shirt, we ask about it. If an adolescent brings a book or is listening to music, we ask them to describe the book or song. The point is not to make an aesthetic judgment about the stuffed animals, clothes, books, or music with which a young person presents but to understand how that person thinks.

Asking about something that the patient is consciously (or unconsciously) presenting to you also builds the therapeutic alliance. Imagine if you walked into a medical encounter and your physician began telling you about their interests but waved off any attempts to discuss your own. You, like most of us, would feel ignored and would likely be reluctant to engage in treatment with the physician. Now imagine if you visited another physician and they knew your name, said it correctly, and then asked how you came by your name. You would likely be more engaged with this second physician and their treatment. You can (and should) extend the same engaging courtesy to the children and adolescents you meet as patients.

We favor beginning every interview by introducing yourself, asking the young person their name, assessing their expectations for the encounter, clarifying any misperceptions, and giving a sense of how long the encounter will last. Caregivers, rather than young people themselves, set up most evaluations, so verbally acknowledging this right away (*"So, your mom wanted you to see me…."*) shows a young person that you can see things through their eyes.

We believe that when the encounter is limited to 30 minutes, you can successfully develop a therapeutic alliance and perform a diagnostic interview, with a few caveats.

- Any psychiatric examination that obtains all the information from a single source is incomplete. This is especially true when you are interviewing a child or an adolescent. You should disclose to the person you are interviewing that you will be speaking to some of their adult caregivers about their health and what you will be discussing. See Chapter 4, "Working Together on Common Clinical Concerns," and Chapter 11, "Using DSM-5-TR Assessment Measures to Aid Diagnosis," for tools to use in interviewing adult caregivers.

- A successful psychiatric examination ultimately provides access to the internal world of a person. The thoughts, impulses, and desires of a young person can be engaged in many ways. In what follows, we offer an interview best suited for a young person who can tolerate direct questions. When you are interviewing a child or an adolescent who cannot do so because of age, impairment, or disinterest, we recommend focusing on the most essential portion of the examination and spending the remainder of your time developing a therapeutic alliance.
- A skilled psychiatric examination always includes an account of the relationships that constitute a person's existence. This is especially true with children and adolescents, whose dependence on other people is more apparent than it is for the average adult. During every interview with a young person, we always ask questions such as *"Who do you live with?"* *"How do you spend your days?"* *"Who cares for you?"* and *"Who can you trust?"* These kinds of questions naturally lead into other critical questions about the caregivers in a young person's life.

With these caveats in mind, we offer the following as a guideline for a diagnostic interview that uses DSM-5-TR (American Psychiatric Association 2022) criteria. The interview does not include prompts for DSM-5-TR categories that are uncommon in childhood and adolescence—namely, the neurocognitive, gambling, paraphilia, personality, and sexual dysfunction disorders. (We do, however, provide guidance in Chapter 11 for using the Personality Inventory for DSM-5 to assess personality traits.) We have taught a version of this interview to students, residents, fellows, and faculty. Until you develop the habits of an experienced practitioner, it helps to practice a structured interview. This helps in becoming comfortable asking about intimate concerns, remembering to screen all patients for the major categories of mental illness, and developing good interview habits.

Of course, using a structured interview has a downside. We have sometimes witnessed practitioners read one question after another, without stopping for the usual pauses that signify human speech or even looking at the patient. In *The Pocket Guide to the DSM-5-TR® Diagnostic Exam* (Nussbaum 2022), we called these kinds of interviewers psychiatric robots who ask things like *"I hear you are suicidal, but can you spell* world *backward?"*—questions that show more fidelity to an outlined interview than attention to the specific person before them. These kinds of interviewers speak so stiffly and stay so determinedly on script that when witnessing them, you wonder which of their joints need to be oiled first. We both have performed the psychiatric robot interview ourselves at some point during our careers. We wrote this guide in part so that you can learn from our mistakes.

What we have found (and still find) challenging is providing the right amount of structure for the interview. An excitable person needs calm, a sad person needs encouragement, and sometimes the same person needs both in the same interview. Fortunately, you always have the best possible guide: the person before you. Follow their lead. Observe their body language. If they appear disinterested, it is time to alter your approach.

As you use this diagnostic interview, strike a balance between becoming a psychiatric robot and practicing a formal version until it becomes a habit. The 30-minute diagnostic interview will seem forced at first, but gradually it provides the infrastructure for a conversational interview.

No matter how distracted or upset the patient, good interviewers always give the person a few minutes to speak their own mind. Then, they summarize and clarify the patient's concerns and organize the examination as necessary, modulating the structure and language of the interview to fit the needs of the patient. They ask clear and succinct questions. If the patient is vague, they seek precision. If the patient remains vague, they explore why. They do not ask permission to change the subject but use transition statements, such as "*I think I understand this, but how about that?*" Developing a supply of stock questions is helpful, which is why we advise using this structured interview until it becomes a habit. Then you can use these questions to develop a conversational style for an interview in which a patient tells their story, you form an alliance with them, you gain insight into their thought process, and you gather the clinical data needed to make an accurate diagnosis. When you do so, you reduce the patient's alienation by making the strange more familiar.

Outline of the 30-Minute Pediatric Diagnostic Interview

The interview outline in this section includes headings that indicate the time allotted for each portion of the interview (**boldface** type), instructions for the interviewer (roman type), and questions for the interviewer to ask (*italic* type).

Minute 1

Introduce yourself to the patient. Ask how they would like to be addressed. Set expectations for how long you will meet and what you will accomplish. Describe applicable limits of confidentiality with an adolescent, such as *"What we talk about will remain confidential except if there is a risk for your safety—then we will talk together with your parent about how to best keep you safe."* Then ask, *"Why are you here today?"*

Minutes 2–4

Listen

A patient's uninterrupted speech indicates much of their mental status, guides your history taking, and builds the alliance. As they speak, listen to the content and form of their statements. What are they saying or not saying? How are they saying it? How do their statements match their appearance? Although you may be tempted to interrupt or begin asking questions, with experience you will find that allowing the person to talk initially without interruptions gives you more information about them than the answers to your questions will. When you do speak next, try to have your question be both responsive and open-ended, along the lines of *"You said ____; can you tell me more about that?"* Depending on the nature of the illness, some people will be unable to fill this time; their inability to do so reveals valuable information about their mental status and distress. When a person does not speak spontaneously, you may have to use prompts and proceed to the history of the current illness. Remember: the clinician who is silent at first is often heard afterward.

Minutes 5–12

History of the Current Illness

Your questions should follow the DSM-5 criteria, as described in Chapter 7, "Reaching a DSM-5-TR Pediatric Diagnosis When You Have 45 Minutes or More." In addition, you should focus on what has changed recently—the "Why now?" of the presentation. As you do, seek understanding of precipitating events by asking questions like the following: *"When did your current distress begin? When was the last time you felt emotionally well? Can you identify any precipitating, perpetuating, or extenuating events? How have your thoughts and behaviors affected your ability to function with family, friends, and your community? How do you view your current level of functioning, and how is it different from what it was days, weeks, or months ago?"*

Psychiatric History

"When did you first notice symptoms? When did you first seek treatment? Did you ever experience a full recovery? Have you ever been hospitalized? How many times? What was the reason for those hospitalizations, and how long were you hospitalized? Do you receive outpatient mental health treatment? Do you take medications for a mental illness? Which medicines have helped the most? Did you have any adverse effects from any medications? What was the reason for stopping any prior medications? How long were you taking each medication, and how often did you take it? Do you know the name, strength, and number of doses per day of medicines you are currently taking?"

Safety

Some clinicians feel uncomfortable asking safety questions, worrying that they will upset patients or even give them ideas about ways to hurt themselves or others. These fears are largely unfounded, and with practice you will find that these questions become easier to ask. They are always essential for an overall risk assessment. *"Do you frequently think about hurting yourself? Have you ever hurt yourself, such as cutting or hitting? Have you ever attempted to kill yourself? How many attempts have you made? What did you do? What medical or psychiatric treatment did you receive after these attempts? Do you often become so upset that you make or even act on verbal threats to hurt other people, animals, or property? Have you ever been aggressive to people or animals, destroyed property, tricked other people, or stolen things?"*

Minutes 13–17

Review of Systems

The psychiatric review of systems is a brief overview of common psychiatric symptoms that you may not have elicited in the history of the current illness. If a person answers affirmatively to these questions, you should explore further with the DSM-5-TR criteria, as modeled in Chapter 7.

Mood. *"Have you been feeling sad, empty, or irritable? Have you lost interest in, or do you get less pleasure from, the things you used to enjoy? Are you angry most of the time? Has there been a time when for many days straight your mood was super happy, you were more self-confident, and you had much more energy than usual? If so, can you describe what happened?"* (See "Depressive Disorders" or "Bipolar and Related Disorders" in Chapter 7.)

Psychosis. *"Have you seen visions or other things that other people did not see? Have you heard noises, sounds, or voices that other people did not hear? Do you ever feel like people are following you or trying to hurt you in some way? Have you ever felt that you had special powers, such as reading other people's minds? While watching videos or listening to music, have you ever felt that it was referring just to you?"* (See "Schizophrenia Spectrum and Other Psychotic Disorders" in Chapter 7.)

Anxiety. *"Would you say that you worry a lot or more than other kids your age? Do people say that you worry too much or are too shy? Do you feel afraid when you're alone or away from your family? Do you get scared about going to school? Is it hard for you to control or stop your worrying? Are there specific things, places, or situations that make you feel very anxious or fearful? Have you ever felt suddenly frightened, nervous, or anxious for no reason at all? If so, can you tell me about that?"* (See "Anxiety Disorders" in Chapter 7.)

Obsessions and compulsions. *"Do you frequently experience intrusive and unwanted images, thoughts, or urges? Are there any physical acts that you feel like you must do to avoid or reduce the distress associated with these images, thoughts, or urges?"* (See "Obsessive-Compulsive and Related Disorders" in Chapter 7.)

Trauma. *"What is the worst thing that has ever happened to you? Has someone ever touched you in a way you did not want? Have you ever felt that your life was in danger or thought that you were going to be seriously injured? Do you have unhappy memories that make it hard to sleep or to feel OK now?"* (See "Trauma- and Stressor-Related Disorders" in Chapter 7.)

Dissociation. *"Do people say that you daydream a lot or look spaced out? Do you lose track of time and feel unsure of what you did during that time? Do you ever feel as if you are standing outside* *your body or watching yourself?"* (See "Dissociative Disorders" in Chapter 7.)

Eating and feeding. *"What do you think of your appearance? Do you avoid particular foods so much that it negatively affects your health or weight? Do you worry about losing control over how much you eat?"* (See "Feeding and Eating Disorders" in Chapter 7.)

Elimination. *"Have you had any problem with leaking urine or feces onto your clothing or bed?"* (See "Elimination Disorders" in Chapter 7.)

Somatic concerns. *"Do you worry about your health more than other kids do? Do you often miss school because you do not feel well? Do you get sick with aches and pains more often than most young people do?"* (See "Somatic Symptom and Related Disorders" in Chapter 7.)

Sleeping. *"Do you struggle to fall asleep, or do you wake up a lot at night? Do you often feel sleepy during the day? Has anyone said that you stop breathing or gasp for air while sleeping?"* (See "Sleep-Wake Disorders" in Chapter 7.)

Substances and other addictions. *"In the past year, have you drunk alcohol, smoked marijuana, or used anything else to get high? Have you ever ridden in a car with someone who was high or drinking alcohol? Do you ever use alcohol or drugs when you are alone? Do you ever use alcohol or drugs to relax?"* (Knight et al. 2002). (See "Substance-Related and Addictive Disorders" in Chapter 7.)

Minutes 18–23
Past Medical History

"Do you have any chronic medical problems? Have these illnesses affected you emotionally? Have you ever undergone surgery? Have you ever experienced a seizure or hit your head so hard that you lost consciousness? Do you take any medications for medical illness? Do you take any supplements, vitamins, or over-the-counter or herbal medicines regularly?"

Allergies. *"Are you allergic to any medications?"* If so: *"Can you describe your allergy?"*

Family history. *"Have any of your relatives ever had nervousness, a nervous breakdown, depression, mania, psychosis or schizophrenia, problems resulting from excessive drinking or drug abuse;*

made suicide attempts; or required psychiatric hospitalization? Have any of your first-degree relatives died by suicide?"

Developmental history. *"Do you know if your mother had any difficulties during her pregnancy or delivery? What were you like as a young child? Did you ever receive developmental, speech, or special education services?"* (See Chapter 13, "Recognizing Developmental Red Flags," for early developmental milestones.) Look at the child's current height and weight on a growth curve. If applicable, ask "When did you reach puberty, and how did you feel about it?"*

Social history. *"Did you have any behavior or learning problems during your early childhood? When you started school, did you have trouble relating socially to your classmates or difficulty keeping up academically? How far have you made it in school? Who lived in your home during your early childhood? Who lives there now? Was a religious faith part of your upbringing? Is it currently? Have you ever held a job outside of the home? Have you ever been suspended? Expelled? Arrested? Jailed? What do you like to do? How do you spend your time online? What do you like about yourself? What do your friends like about you? Do you have any friends you can confide in? Are you sexually active? Are you really uncomfortable with your assigned gender?"*

Minutes 24–28

Mental Status Examination

You have already observed or obtained most of the pertinent mental status examination data, but now is the opportunity to organize your findings so you can address any remaining components. A detailed version of the resulting mental status examination is in Chapter 10, "Organizing a Comprehensive Pediatric Mental Status Examination With a Psychiatric Glossary," but the essential components include the following:

- Appearance
- Behavior
- Speech
- Emotion
- Thought process
- Thought content
- Cognition and intellectual resources
- Insight and judgment: *"What problems do you have? Are you sick in any way? What are your future plans?"*

Mini-Mental State Examination

The Mini-Mental State Examination (MMSE) is an assessment of basic cognitive ability commonly used in adult and geriatric psychiatric care that has standardized questions and yields a numerical score. We find that the MMSE is less pertinent to young persons than to older adults. When it is used, the MMSE is more challenging to interpret for patients of younger developmental ages. However, if a major mental illness (e.g., schizophrenia) or encephalopathy is suspected, the MMSE may add diagnostic value. When the MMSE is used, the lead-in could be along the lines of *"Have you had any problems with your concentration or your memory? Can you help me understand the extent to which you might be having those types of difficulties?"* The MMSE includes the following items: name, date and time, place, immediate recall, attention (counting backward from 100 by sevens, spelling *world* backward), delayed recall, general information (president, governor, five large cities), abstractions, proverbs, naming, repetition, three-stage command, reading, copying, and writing (Folstein et al. 1975).

Minutes 29–30

Ask any follow-up questions. Thank the patient for their time and, if appropriate, begin discussing diagnosis and treatment. Consider asking the following: *"Have the questions I asked addressed your major concerns? Is there anything important I missed or anything that I really should know about to better understand what you are going through?"*

PART II

Engaging Children and Adolescents With DSM-5-TR

Chapter 7

Reaching a DSM-5-TR Pediatric Diagnosis When You Have 45 Minutes or More

In Chapter 6, "Reaching a DSM-5-TR Diagnosis When You Have 30 Minutes," we outlined a diagnostic interview that included a screening question for each of the DSM-5-TR (American Psychiatric Association 2022) categories of mental disorders commonly experienced by children and adolescents. If you are speaking with a young person who answers affirmatively to one of those questions, the screening questions are the avenues of the psychiatric diagnostic interview. A good interviewer skillfully travels these avenues with the young person and, when possible, reaches a specific and accurate diagnosis along the way. In this chapter, we set aside any external time limitations you might otherwise experience in your diagnostic interview process and simply describe a process for evaluating a young person that follows DSM-5-TR diagnostic criteria.

This chapter follows the order of DSM-5-TR diagnostic classes in the primary text, beginning with neurodevelopmental disorders. For each diagnostic class presented, whether bipolar and related disorders or elimination disorders, the section begins with one or more screening questions from the model interview presented in Chapter 6. After the screening questions, there can be follow-up questions. If the follow-up questions include a measure of impairment or a measure of time, these measures are a required part of the subsequent diagnostic criteria. By asking follow-up questions before the additional symptom questions in the diagnostic criteria, we make the interview more efficient and precise while reserving the full diagnosis of a mental disorder for a person impaired by their experiences.

The screening and follow-up questions are followed by the diagnostic criteria. When the diagnostic criteria are to be elicited by the interviewer, we offer *italicized* prompts for the relevant symptom. We structured these questions so that an affirmative answer meets the criteria for that symptom. When the diagnostic criteria are observed rather than elicited, as in the case of disorganized speech, psychomotor retardation, or autonomic hyperactivity, they are listed as instructions to the interviewer, set in roman type. The minimum number of symptoms necessary to reach a particular diagnosis is underlined. We do not list all the possible questions that can be used to elicit a relevant symptom, but these questions are specifically designed to follow DSM-5-TR. To make the diagnostic process as clear as possible, we have included negative criteria for a DSM-5-TR diagnosis under the heading "Exclusion(s)." For example, according to DSM-5-TR, a young person's recurrent, aggressive outbursts do not meet criteria for intermittent explosive disorder if they occur only during an adjustment disorder. These exclusion criteria usually do not require you to ask a specific question but instead depend on the history you elicit. The most common subtypes, specifiers, and severity measures are listed under the heading "Modifiers," but the complete array of modifiers is found only in DSM-5-TR.

In the interest of brevity, this guide includes diagnostic questions for the most common DSM-5-TR disorders. The idea is to focus on the diagnostic criteria for the paradigmatic disorders in each section before exploring the related diagnoses—that is, to follow the main streets of DSM-5-TR before traveling its side streets.

In this book, the side streets are labeled *alternatives*, a term that is not used in DSM-5-TR. These alternatives include only related diagnoses from the same DSM-5-TR chapter. For example, schizophreniform disorder is listed as an alternative to schizophrenia because both are grouped together in DSM-5-TR. In contrast, bipolar I disorder and other diagnoses listed in the differential diagnosis for schizophrenia are not in the alternatives section for schizophrenia because these disorders are found in different sections of DSM-5-TR. For each diagnosis listed as an alternative, the essential diagnostic criteria are included, and the interviewer is referred to the corresponding pages in DSM-5-TR to read the diagnostic criteria and associated material in detail. We include all DSM-5-TR diagnoses, and we have eliminated repetitive criteria, especially for the various mental disorders associated with another medical condition or substance-induced mental disorders, in which, broadly, the symptoms of a disorder are present as a direct effect of another medical condition or the use of a substance.

As this overview suggests, this book is no substitute for DSM-5-TR but is a practical diagnostic tool with specific phrasing you can use, an operationalized version of DSM-5-TR—the equivalent of the sketched version of a city street that a phone's map displays rather than a detailed portrait of each side street. This book helps you reach your destination in a timely fashion and then invites you into the details of DSM-5-TR.

Neurodevelopmental Disorders

DSM-5-TR pp. 35–99

This section contains questions phrased for interviewing an older child with an ability to self-reflect. For younger children, rephrase these questions to interview the child's caregiver instead.

Screening questions: *Did you have any learning problems, or did you get into trouble a lot for your behavior when you were younger? When you started school, did you have trouble getting along with your classmates or difficulty keeping up academically?*

If yes, ask: *Do you have trouble concentrating or struggle with being impulsive or overactive? Do you have difficulty communicating with other people? Are there specific things that you do frequently and find hard to control? Do you struggle to learn, more than your classmates do?*

- If deficits in intellectual functioning or specific academic skills predominate, proceed to intellectual disability (intellectual developmental disorder) criteria.
- If deficits in social interactions or impairing motor behaviors predominate, proceed to autism spectrum disorder criteria.
- If inattention, hyperactivity, or impulsivity predominate, proceed to attention-deficit/hyperactivity disorder (ADHD) criteria.

1. Intellectual Developmental Disorder (Intellectual Disability)

a. Inclusion: Requires intellectual deficits, beginning during early development, that impair adaptive function as manifested by <u>both</u> of the following symptoms.

 i. Deficits in intellectual functions, such as reasoning, problem-solving, planning, abstract thinking, judgment, academic learning, and experiential learning. Must be confirmed by both clinical assessment and individualized, standardized intelligence testing.

 ii. Impaired adaptive functioning, normalized for age and culture, that restricts participation and performance in one or more aspects of daily life activities. The limitations result in the need for ongoing support at school, at work, or for independent life.

b. Modifiers

 i. Severity (see DSM-5-TR, pp. 39–41, Table 1)

 • Mild
 • Moderate
 • Severe
 • Profound

c. Alternatives

 i. If a person younger than 5 years fails to meet expected developmental milestones in several areas of intellectual functioning and is unable to undergo systematic assessment of intellectual functioning, consider global developmental delay (see DSM-5-TR, p. 46), a diagnosis that requires reassessment after a period of time.

 ii. If a person older than 5 years exhibits intellectual disability that cannot be well characterized because of associated sensory or physical impairments, consider unspecified intellectual developmental disorder (see DSM-5-TR, p. 46). This diagnosis should be used only in exceptional circumstances and requires eventual reassessment.

 iii. If a person has persistent difficulties in the acquisition of language (spoken, written, sign, or other modalities) that begin in the early developmental period and result in substantial functional limitations, consider the diagnosis of language disorder (full criteria are available in DSM-5-TR, p. 47).

Language disorder occurs as a primary impairment or coexists with other disorders. This diagnosis should not be used if the language difficulties are better explained by hearing or sensory impairment, intellectual disability, or global developmental delay or are caused by another medical or neurological condition.

iv. If a person has persistent difficulties in speech sound production that interfere with speech intelligibility or prevent verbal communication of messages, consider speech sound disorder (full criteria are available in DSM-5-TR, p. 50). The symptoms must be present in the early developmental period and result in limitations in effective communication, social participation, academic achievement, and occupational performance, individually or in any combination. Speech sound disorder occurs as a primary impairment or coexists with other disorders or congenital or acquired conditions. This diagnosis should not be used if the speech sound difficulties are due to congenital or acquired medical or neurological conditions.

v. If a person has marked and frequent disturbances in the fluency and time patterning of speech that are inappropriate for the person's age and language skills, consider childhood-onset fluency disorder (stuttering) (full criteria are available in DSM-5-TR, pp. 51–52). Symptoms must begin in the early developmental period. The disturbance must cause anxiety about speaking or the ability to communicate effectively. The disorder can co-exist with other disorders. However, the diagnosis should not be used if the disorder is attributable to a speech-motor or sensory deficit, is due to another medical or neurological condition, or is better explained by another mental disorder.

vi. If a person has persistent difficulties in the social use of verbal and nonverbal communication that functionally limit effective communication, social participation, social relationships, academic achievement, or occupational performance, consider social (pragmatic) communication disorder (full criteria are available in DSM-5-TR, p. 54). Symptoms begin during the early developmental period. The disorder can coexist with other disorders. However, this diagnosis should not be used if the symptoms are better explained by intellectual disability, global developmental delay, or another mental disorder or are attributable to another medical or neurological condition.

  vii. If a person has symptoms of a communication disorder that cause clinically significant distress or impairment but do not meet the full criteria for a communication disorder or another neurodevelopmental disorder, consider unspecified communication disorder (see DSM-5-TR, p. 56).

  viii. If a person has persistent difficulties in learning and using academic skills that begin during the school-age years and eventually result in significant interference with academic or occupational performance, consider specific learning disorder (full criteria, along with severity ratings, are available in DSM-5-TR, pp. 76–78). To meet criteria, the current skills must be well below the average range for the person's age, gender, cultural group, and level of education. The symptoms must not be better accounted for by another intellectual, medical, mental, neurological, or sensory disorder.

2. Autism Spectrum Disorder

This section contains questions phrased for interviewing an older child with an ability to self-reflect. For younger children or those with limited cognitive functioning, rephrase these questions to interview the child's caregiver instead.

  a. Inclusion: Requires persistent deficits in social communication and social interaction, across multiple contexts, that are present in early childhood but that may not manifest until social demands exceed limited capacities and that cause clinically significant impairment in functioning. The disorder is marked by <u>all</u> of the following persistent deficits in social communication and interaction.

    i. Deficits in social-emotional reciprocity: *When you meet someone, how do you introduce yourself? Do you find it hard to greet another person? Do you find it hard to share your interests, thoughts, and feelings with other people? Do you dislike to hear about what other people are interested in or how they feel?*

ii. Deficits in nonverbal communicative behaviors used for social interaction; these are usually observed by a practitioner and range from poorly integrated verbal and nonverbal communication, to abnormalities in eye contact and body language or deficits in understanding and using nonverbal communication, to a total lack of facial expression or gestures.

iii. Deficits in developing and maintaining relationships: *Are you disinterested in other people? Are you unable to engage in imaginative play with other people? Do you find it difficult to make new friends? When a situation changes, do you find it hard to adjust what you do in response?*

b. Inclusion: In addition, the diagnosis requires at least <u>two</u> of the following signs of restricted, repetitive patterns of behavior, interests, or activities.

i. Stereotyped or repetitive speech, motor movements, or use of objects, such as simple motor stereotypies, echolalia, repetitive use of objects, or idiosyncratic phrases.

ii. Insistence on sameness and excessive adherence to routines or avoidance of change: *Do you have any special routines or patterns of behavior? What happens when you cannot follow these routines or engage in these behaviors? Do you struggle to change?*

iii. Restricted interests of abnormal intensity or focus: *Do you intensely focus on, or find yourself very interested in, just a few things?*

iv. Hyper- or hyporreactivity to sensory input: *How do you experience something that is painful? Something hot? Something cold? Are there particular sounds, textures, or smells to which you respond strongly? Do you find yourself fascinated with lights or spinning objects?*

c. Modifiers

i. Specifiers

- With (or without) accompanying intellectual impairment
- With (or without) accompanying language impairment
- Associated with a known medical or genetic condition or environmental factor

- Associated with another neurodevelopmental, mental, or behavioral disorder
- With catatonia

ii. Severity is coded separately for the social communication impairments and for the restricted, repetitive patterns of behavior.

- Level 1: Requiring support
- Level 2: Requiring substantial support
- Level 3: Requiring very substantial support

d. Alternatives

i. If a person exhibits coordinated motor performance substantially below expected levels that significantly interferes with activities of daily living or academic achievement and that began in the early developmental period, consider developmental coordination disorder (full criteria are in DSM-5-TR, pp. 85–86). Examples include clumsiness as well as slow and inaccurate performance of motor skills. The disturbance cannot be due to another medical or neurological condition or be better explained by another mental disorder.

ii. If a person exhibits repetitive, seemingly driven, yet apparently purposeless motor behavior, such as hand shaking or waving, body rocking, head banging, or self-biting, consider stereotypic movement disorder (full criteria are in DSM-5-TR, p. 89). The motor disturbance causes clinically significant distress or impairment. The motor behavior is not due to the direct physiological effects of a substance or a general medical condition and is not better explained by the symptoms of another mental disorder.

iii. A tic is a sudden, rapid, recurrent, nonrhythmic motor movement or vocalization. If a person experiences both motor and vocal tics beginning before age 18 years, consider Tourette's disorder (full criteria are in DSM-5-TR, p. 93). The tics may wax and wane in frequency but must persist for at least 1 year after onset. The tics cannot be due to the direct physiological effects of another medical condition or a substance.

iv. If a person experiences either motor or vocal tics, but not both, during the illness, and has never had symptoms that have met criteria for Tourette's disorder, consider persistent (chronic) motor or vocal tic disorder (full criteria are in DSM-5-TR, p. 93). The onset is before age 18 years, and the tics may wax and wane in frequency but must have persisted for more than 1 year since their onset.

v. If a person experiences motor and/or vocal tics for at least 1 year, beginning before age 18 years, and the tics are not due to the direct physiological consequences of another medical condition or substance, and the person has never had symptoms that have met criteria for Tourette's disorder, consider persistent (chronic) motor or vocal tic disorder (full criteria are in DSM-5-TR, p. 93). The tics may wax and wane in frequency but must have persisted for more than 1 year since their onset.

vi. If a person experiences motor and/or vocal tics for less than 1 year, beginning before age 18 years, and the tics are not attributable to the physiological consequences of a substance or another medical condition, and the criteria for Tourette's disorder or persistent (chronic) motor or vocal tic disorder have never been met, consider provisional tic disorder (full criteria are in DSM-5-TR, p. 93).

vii. If a person experiences tics that do not meet criteria for a specific tic disorder because the movements or vocalizations are atypical in relation to age at onset or clinical presentation, consider other specified tic disorder or unspecified tic disorder (see DSM-5-TR, p. 98).

3. Attention-Deficit/Hyperactivity Disorder

a. Inclusion: Requires a pattern of behavior, with onset before age 12 years, that is present in multiple settings and gives rise to difficulties in social, educational, or work performance. The symptoms must be persistently present for at least 6 months to a degree inconsistent with the person's developmental level. The disorder is manifested by at least six of the following symptoms of inattention.

i. Overlooks details: *Over at least the past 6 months, have other people told you that you often overlook or miss details or that you made careless mistakes in your work?*

ii. Task inattention: *Do you often have difficulty staying focused on a task or activity, such as reading a lengthy piece of writing or listening to a lecture or conversation?*

iii. Appears not to listen: *Do other people tell you that when they speak to you, your mind often seems to be elsewhere or it seems like you are not listening?*

iv. Fails to finish tasks: *Do you often struggle to finish schoolwork, chores, or work assignments because you lose focus or are easily sidetracked?*

v. Difficulty organizing tasks: *Do you often find it difficult to organize tasks or activities? Do you struggle with time management or fail to meet deadlines?*

vi. Avoids tasks requiring sustained mental activity: *Do you often avoid tasks that require sustained mental effort?*

vii. Often loses things necessary for tasks: *Do you often lose things that are essential for tasks or activities, such as school materials, books, tools, wallets, keys, paperwork, eyeglasses, or your phone?*

viii. Easily distracted: *Do you find that you are often easily distracted by things or thoughts unrelated to the activity or task you are supposed to be doing?*

ix. Often forgetful: *Do you find, or do other people find, that you are often forgetful in your daily activities?*

b. Inclusion: Alternatively, requires the presence of at least six of the following manifestations of hyperactivity and impulsivity over the same course.

i. Fidgets: *Over the past 6 months, have you often found yourself fidgeting with your hands or feet? Do you find it hard to sit without squirming?*

ii. Leaves seat: *When you are in a situation where you are expected to sit, do you often leave your seat?*

iii. Runs or climbs: *Do you often find yourself running around or climbing in a situation where doing so is inappropriate?*

iv. Unable to maintain quiet: *Do you often find yourself unable to play or work quietly?*

v. Hyperactivity: *Do you often feel as if you are, or do other people describe you as always being, "on the go" or as acting as if you were "driven by a motor"? Do you find it uncomfortable to sit still for an extended time?*

vi. Talks excessively: *Do you often talk excessively?*

vii. Blurts answers: *Do you often struggle to wait your*

turn in a conversation? Do you often complete other people's sentences or blurt out an answer before a question has been completed?

viii. Struggles to take turns: *Do you often have difficulty waiting your turn or waiting in line?*

ix. Interrupts or intrudes: *Do you often butt into other people's activities, conversations, or games? Do you often start using other people's things without permission?*

c. Exclusion: If the criteria are not met in two or more settings, or there is no evidence that the symptoms interfere with functioning, the symptoms occur only in the context of a psychotic disorder, or the symptoms are better explained by another mental disorder (e.g., an anxiety disorder causing inattention), do not make the diagnosis.

d. Modifiers

i. Specifiers

- Combined presentation: If both inattention and hyperactivity-impulsivity criteria are met for the past 6 months.
- Predominantly inattentive presentation: If inattention criteria are met but hyperactivity-impulsivity criteria have not been met for the past 6 months.
- Predominantly hyperactive/impulsive presentation: If hyperactivity-impulsivity criteria are met and inattention criteria have not been met for the past 6 months.
- In partial remission if full criteria no longer met but still symptomatic.

ii. Severity

- Mild: Few, if any, symptoms in excess of those required to make the diagnosis are present, and symptoms result in no more than minor impairments in social or occupational functioning.
- Moderate: Symptoms or functional impairment between "mild" and "severe" are present.
- Severe: Many symptoms in excess of those required to make the diagnosis, or several symptoms that are particularly severe, are present, or the symptoms result in marked impairment in social or occupational functioning.

e. Alternative: If a young person is experiencing sub-threshold symptoms or you have not yet had sufficient opportunity to verify all criteria, consider other specified attention-deficit/hyperactivity disorder or unspecified attention-deficit/hyperactivity disorder (see DSM-5-TR, p. 76). The symptoms must be associated with impairment, must not occur exclusively during the course of schizophrenia or another psychotic disorder, and must not be better explained by another mental disorder.

Schizophrenia Spectrum and Other Psychotic Disorders

DSM-5-TR pp. 101–138

Screening questions: *Have you seen visions or other things that other people did not see? Have you heard noises, sounds, or voices that other people did not hear? Do you ever feel like people are following you or trying to hurt you in some way? Have you ever felt that you had special powers, such as reading other people's minds? While watching videos or listening to music, have you ever felt that it was referring just to you?*

If yes, ask: *Do these experiences influence your behavior or tell you to do things? Did these experiences ever cause you significant trouble with your friends or family, at school, or in another setting?*

- If yes, proceed to schizophrenia criteria.

1. Schizophrenia

    a. Inclusion: Requires at least 6 months of continuous signs of disturbance, which may include prodromal or residual symptoms. During at least 1 month of that period, at least <u>two</u> of the following symptoms are present, and at least <u>one</u> of the symptoms must be delusions, hallucinations, or disorganized speech.

        i. Delusions: *Is anyone working to harm or hurt you? When you read a book, watch television, or use a computer, do you ever find that there are messages intended just for you? Do you have special powers or abilities?*

        ii. Hallucinations: *When you are awake, do you ever hear a voice different from your own thoughts that other peo-*

ple cannot hear? When you are awake, do you ever see things that other people cannot see?

    iii. Disorganized speech like frequent derailment or incoherence

    iv. Grossly disorganized or catatonic behavior

    v. Negative symptoms such as diminished emotional expression or avolition

b. Exclusions

    i. If the disturbance is attributable to the physiological effects of a substance (e.g., a drug of abuse, a medication) or another medical condition, do not make the diagnosis.

    ii. If a young person has been diagnosed with an autism spectrum disorder or a communication disorder of childhood onset, schizophrenia may be diagnosed only if prominent delusions or hallucinations are also present for at least 1 month.

c. Modifiers

    i. Specifiers

- First episode, currently in acute episode
- First episode, currently in partial remission
- First episode, currently in full remission
- Multiple episodes, currently in acute episode
- Multiple episodes, currently in partial remission
- Multiple episodes, currently in full remission
- Continuous
- Unspecified

    ii. Additional specifiers

- With catatonia: Use when at least <u>three</u> of the following are present: stupor, catalepsy, waxy flexibility, mutism, negativism, posturing, mannerisms, stereotypies, agitation, grimacing, echolalia, echopraxia.

    iii. Severity

- Severity is rated by a quantitative assessment of the primary symptoms of psychosis, each of which may be rated for its current severity on a 5-point scale (see Clinician-Rated Dimensions of Psychosis Symptom Severity in DSM-5-TR, pp. 851–853).

d. Alternatives

    i. If a person experiences only delusions, whether bizarre or nonbizarre, and has functioning that is not markedly impaired beyond the ramifications of their delusion, consider delusional disorder (full criteria are in DSM-5-TR, pp. 104–106). The criteria include multiple specifiers: erotomanic, grandiose, jealous, persecutory, and somatic. If a person has ever had symptoms that have met full criteria for schizophrenia, if the delusions occur during catatonia, if the delusions are due to the physiological effects of a substance or another medical condition, or if the delusions are better explained by another mental disorder, do not make the diagnosis.

    ii. If a person has experienced at least 1 day but less than 1 month of schizophrenia symptoms, consider brief psychotic disorder (full criteria are in DSM-5-TR, pp. 108–109). The person usually experiences an acute onset with emotional turmoil or overwhelming confusion. The person exhibits fewer negative symptoms, experiences less functional impairment, and always experiences an eventual return to their previous level of functioning.

    iii. If a person has experienced at least 1 month but less than 6 months of schizophrenia symptoms, consider schizophreniform disorder (full criteria are in DSM-5-TR, pp. 111–112). This diagnosis should not be used if the disturbance is due to the physiological effects of a substance or another medical condition.

    iv. If a person whose symptoms meet criteria for schizophrenia also experiences major mood disturbances—either major depressive episodes or manic episodes—for at least half the time their symptoms meet criteria for schizophrenia, consider schizoaffective disorder (full criteria are in DSM-5-TR, pp. 121–122). Over the person's lifetime, they must have experienced at least 2 weeks of delusions or hallucinations in the absence of a major mood episode.

    v. If a substance or medication directly causes delusions and/or hallucinations during substance intoxication or withdrawal, consider substance/medication-induced psychotic disorder (full criteria are in DSM-5-TR, pp. 126–127) while remembering that roughly one-third of people diagnosed with substance-induced psychotic disorder eventually develop schizophrenia spectrum or bipolar disorders when followed longitudinally. The criteria include multiple specifiers for individual substances.

vi. If another medical condition directly causes the psychotic episode, consider psychotic disorder due to another medical condition (full criteria are in DSM-5-TR, p. 131). This diagnosis should be considered when biological plausibility, temporality, and atypical psychotic symptoms are present. This diagnosis should not be used during an episode of delirium or when the psychotic episode is better explained by another mental disorder.

vii. If a person experiences psychotic symptoms that cause clinically significant distress or functional impairment without meeting full criteria for another psychotic disorder, consider unspecified schizophrenia spectrum and other psychotic disorder (see DSM-5-TR, p. 138). If you wish to communicate the specific reason why a person's symptoms do not meet the criteria, consider other specified schizophrenia spectrum and other psychotic disorder (see DSM-5-TR, p. 138). Examples include persistent auditory hallucinations in the absence of any other psychotic symptom and delusional symptoms in the partner of an individual with delusional disorder.

Bipolar and Related Disorders

DSM-5-TR pp. 139–175

Screening questions: *Has there been a time when for many days straight your mood was super happy, you were more self-confident, and you had much more energy than usual?*

If yes, ask: *During those times, did you feel this way all day or most of the day? Did those times ever last at least a week or result in your being hospitalized? Did these periods ever cause you significant trouble with your friends or family, at work, or in another setting?*

- If symptoms lasted a week or caused hospitalization, proceed to bipolar I disorder criteria.
- If not, proceed to bipolar II disorder criteria.

1. Bipolar I Disorder

   a. Inclusion: A manic episode—defined as a distinct period of abnormally and persistently elevated or irritable mood and increased goal-directed activity or energy, lasting at least 1 week and present most of the day—additionally requires at least <u>three</u> of the following symptoms.

      i. Inflated self-esteem or grandiosity: *During that period, did you feel especially confident, as though you could accomplish something extraordinary that you could not have done otherwise?*

      ii. Decreased need for sleep: *During that period, did you notice any change in how much sleep you needed to feel rested? Did you feel rested after less than 3 hours of sleep?*

      iii. More talkative than usual: *During that period, did anyone tell you that you talked more than usual or that it was hard to interrupt you?*

      iv. Flight of ideas: *During that period, were your thoughts racing? Did you have so many ideas that you could not keep up with them?*

      v. Distractibility: *During that period, were you having more trouble than usual focusing? Did you find yourself easily distracted?*

      vi. Increased goal-directed activity: *During that period, how did you spend your time? Did you find yourself much more active than usual?*

      vii. Excessive involvement in activities that have a high potential for painful consequences: *During that period, did you engage in activities that were unusual for you? Did you spend money, use substances, or engage in sexual activities in a way that is unusual for you? Did any of these activities cause trouble for you or someone else?*

   b. Exclusions

      i. The occurrence of manic and major depressive episode(s) is not better explained by schizoaffective disorder, schizophrenia, schizophreniform disorder, delusional disorder, or other specified or unspecified schizophrenia spectrum and other psychotic disorder.

ii. The episode is not due to the physiological effects of a substance or another medical condition. However, a manic episode that both emerges during antidepressant treatment and persists beyond the physiological effect of the treatment meets criteria for bipolar I disorder.

c. Modifiers

   i. Current (or most recent) episode

- Manic
- Hypomanic
- Depressed
- Unspecified (use when the symptoms, but not the duration, of the criteria are met)

  ii. Specifiers

- With anxious distress
- With mixed features: Use if at least <u>three</u> of the symptoms of a major depressive episode are present simultaneously.
- With rapid cycling: Use if a patient experienced at least <u>four</u> episodes (manic, hypomanic, or depressive) in the previous 12 months.
- With melancholic features
- With atypical features
- With mood-congruent psychotic features
- With mood-incongruent psychotic features
- With catatonia
- With peripartum onset: Use if the onset of mood symptoms occurs during pregnancy or in the 4 weeks following delivery.
- With seasonal pattern

 iii. Course and severity

- Current or most recent episode manic, hypomanic, depressed, unspecified

  - Mild
  - Moderate
  - Severe
  - With psychotic features
  - In partial remission

- In full remission
- Unspecified

d. Alternatives

   i. If a substance, including a substance prescribed to treat depression, directly causes the episode, consider substance/medication-induced bipolar and related disorder (full criteria are in DSM-5-TR, pp. 162–163).

   ii. If another medical condition causes the episode, consider bipolar and related disorder due to another medical condition (full criteria are in DSM-5-TR, p. 166).

2. Bipolar II Disorder

a. Inclusion: Requires at least <u>three</u> of the following criteria during a hypomanic episode—defined as a distinct period of abnormally and persistently elevated or irritable mood and increased goal-directed activity or energy, lasting at least 4 days and present most of the day.

   i. Inflated self-esteem or grandiosity: *During that period, did you feel especially confident, as though you could accomplish something extraordinary that you could not have done otherwise?*

   ii. Decreased need for sleep: *During that period, did you notice any change in how much sleep you needed to feel rested? Did you feel rested after less than 3 hours of sleep?*

   iii. More talkative than usual: *During that period, did anyone tell you that you talked more than usual or that it was hard to interrupt you?*

   iv. Flight of ideas: *During that period, were your thoughts racing? Did you have so many ideas that you could not keep up with them?*

   v. Distractibility: *During that period, were you having more trouble than usual focusing? Did you find yourself easily distracted?*

   vi. Increased goal-directed activity: *During that period, how did you spend your time? Did you find yourself much more active than usual?*

   vii. Excessive involvement in activities that have a high potential for painful consequences: *During that period, did you engage in activities that were un-*

usual for you? Did you spend money, use substances, or engage in sexual activities in a way that is unusual for you? Did any of these activities cause trouble for anyone?

b. Exclusions

  i. If there has ever been a manic episode or if the episode is attributable to the physiological effects of a substance or medication, the diagnosis is not given.

  ii. If the hypomanic episode is better explained by schizoaffective disorder, schizophrenia, schizophreniform disorder, delusional disorder, or other specified or unspecified schizophrenia spectrum and other psychotic disorders, the diagnosis is not given.

c. Modifiers

  i. Specify current or most recent episode

   • Hypomanic
   • Depressed

  ii. Specifiers

   • With anxious distress
   • With mixed features: Use if at least <u>three</u> of the symptoms of a major depressive episode are present simultaneously.
   • With rapid cycling
   • With melancholic features
   • With atypical features
   • With mood-congruent psychotic features
   • With mood-incongruent psychotic features
   • With catatonia
   • With peripartum onset
   • With seasonal pattern

  iii. Course

   • In partial remission
   • In full remission

  iv. Severity

   • Mild
   • Moderate
   • Severe

d. Alternatives

    i. If a person reports 1 or more years of multiple hypomanic and depressive symptoms that never rose to the level of a hypomanic or major depressive episode, consider cyclothymic disorder (full criteria are in DSM-5-TR, pp. 159–160). During the same 1-year period, the hypomanic and depressive periods have been present for at least half the time, and the individual has not been without the symptoms for more than 2 months at a time. If the symptoms are due to the physiological effects of a substance or another medical condition, the diagnosis is not given.

    ii. If a person experiences symptoms characteristic of bipolar disorder that cause clinically significant distress or functional impairment without meeting full criteria for a bipolar disorder, consider unspecified bipolar and related disorder (see DSM-5-TR, p. 169). To communicate the specific reason why a person's symptoms do not meet the criteria, as in short-duration hypomania, short-duration cyclothymia, and hypomania without prior major depressive episode, consider other specified bipolar and related disorder (see DSM-5-TR, pp. 168–169). Examples include other short-duration cyclothymia, and hypomanic episode without prior major depressive episode.

Depressive Disorders

DSM-5-TR pp. 177–214

Screening questions: *Have you been feeling sad, empty, or irritable? Have you lost interest in, or do you get less pleasure from, the things you used to enjoy? Are you angry most of the time?*

    If yes, ask: *Did those times ever last at least 2 weeks? Did these periods ever cause you significant trouble with your friends or family, at school, or in another setting?*

- If yes, proceed to major depressive disorder criteria.
- If a child age 6 years or older says no, ask the irritability screening question, which appears after the specifiers for major depressive disorder later in this section.

1. Major Depressive Disorder, Single and Recurrent Episodes

   a. Inclusion: Requires the presence of at least <u>five</u> of the following symptoms, which must include either depressed mood or loss of interest or pleasure (anhedonia), during the same 2-week episode.

      i. Depressed mood most of the day (already assessed)

      ii. Markedly diminished interest or pleasure in activities (already assessed)

      iii. Significant weight loss or gain: *During that period, did you notice any significant change in your appetite? Did you notice any change in your weight?*

      iv. Insomnia or hypersomnia: *During that period, did you find yourself sleeping more or less than usual? Did you have difficulty getting to sleep or staying asleep?*

      v. Psychomotor agitation or retardation: *During that period, did anyone tell you that you seemed to move faster or slower than usual?*

      vi. Fatigue or loss of energy: *During that period, what was your energy level like? Did anyone tell you that you seemed worn down or less energetic than usual?*

      vii. Feelings of worthlessness or excessive guilt: *During that period, did you feel worthless or feel tremendous regret about current or past events or relationships?*

      viii. Diminished concentration: *During that period, were you unable to make decisions or concentrate like you usually do?*

      ix. Recurrent thoughts of death or suicide: *During that period, did you think about death more than you usually do? Did you think about hurting yourself or taking your own life? Did you make a suicide plan?*

   b. Exclusions

      i. If there has ever been a manic episode or a hypomanic episode, or the major depressive episode is attributable to the physiological effects of a substance or to another medical condition, the diagnosis is not given.

      ii. If at least one major depressive episode is better explained by, and superimposed on, schizoaffective disorder, schizophrenia, schizophreniform disorder, delusional disorder, or other specified or unspecified schizophrenia spectrum and other psychotic disorder, the diagnosis is not given.

c. Modifiers

  i. Specifiers

  - With anxious distress
  - With mixed features: Use if at least <u>three</u> of the symptoms of a manic episode are present simultaneously.
  - With melancholic features
  - With atypical features (e.g., mood reactivity, weight gain, hypersomnia, leaden paralysis, long pattern of interpersonal rejection sensitivity)
  - With mood-congruent psychotic features
  - With mood-incongruent psychotic features
  - With catatonia
  - With peripartum onset (during pregnancy or 4 weeks postpartum)
  - With seasonal pattern (onset and remission occur at specific times of the year)

  ii. Course and severity

  - Single episode
  - Recurrent episode
  - In partial remission
  - In full remission
  - Mild
  - Moderate
  - Severe
  - With psychotic features
  - Unspecified

d. Alternatives

  i. If a person reports experiencing depression for at least 2 years resulting in clinically significant distress or impairment, along with at least <u>two</u> additional symptoms of a major depressive episode, consider persistent depressive disorder (full criteria are in DSM-5-TR, pp. 193–194). If a person experiences 2 continuous months without depressive symptoms, do not give the diagnosis. If the person has ever had a manic or hypomanic episode, do not give the diagnosis. If the disturbance is better explained by a psychotic disorder or is due to the physiological effects of a substance or another medical condition, do not give the diagnosis.

ii. If a young woman describes pronounced mood changes that begin in the week before her menses, improve a few days after the onset of menses, and abate in the week after menses, consider premenstrual dysphoric disorder (full criteria are in DSM-5-TR, p. 197). The diagnostic criteria include at least <u>one</u> of the following: marked affective lability, marked irritability or interpersonal conflicts, marked depressed mood, and marked anxiety. At least <u>one</u> of the following symptoms must additionally be present (to reach a total of <u>five</u> symptoms when combined with the symptoms already elicited): decreased interest in usual activities; subjective difficulty concentrating; lethargy, easy fatigability, or marked lack of energy; marked change in appetite; hypersomnia or insomnia; sense of being overwhelmed; and physical symptoms such as breast tenderness or swelling, joint or muscle pain, bloating, and weight gain.

iii. If substance intoxication or withdrawal, including from a medication, directly causes a prominent and persistent depressed mood or anhedonia that occurs outside of delirium, consider a substance/medication-induced depressive disorder (full criteria are in DSM-5-TR, pp. 201–202).

iv. If another medical condition directly causes a prominent and persistent depressed mood or anhedonia that occurs outside of delirium, consider a depressive disorder due to another medical condition (full criteria are in DSM-5-TR, p. 206).

v. If a person experiences a depressive episode that causes clinically significant distress or functional impairment without symptoms that meet full criteria for a depressive disorder, consider unspecified depressive disorder (see DSM-5-TR, p. 210). If you wish to communicate the specific reason why a person's symptoms do not meet the criteria, consider other specified depressive disorder (see DSM-5-TR, pp. 209–210). Examples include recurrent brief depression, short-duration depressive episode, depressive episode with insufficient symptoms, and major depressive disorder super-imposed on a psychotic disorder.

vi. If a person experiences symptoms characteristic of a mood disorder that cause clinically significant distress or impairment without meeting the full criteria for any specific bipolar or depressive disorder, consider unspecified mood disorder (see DSM-5-TR, p. 210). This diagnosis should be considered when it is difficult to choose, as in acute agitation, between unspecified bipolar and depressive disorder.

Irritability screening question for children: *Do you ever lose your temper, yell, or act out?*

If yes, ask: *Do you lose your temper every day or every other day? Does your temper or yelling cause trouble at home or school?*

- If yes, proceed to disruptive mood dysregulation disorder criteria.
- If no, seek collateral information from caregivers or proceed to another diagnostic category.

2. Disruptive Mood Dysregulation Disorder

a. Inclusion: Requires severe recurrent temper outbursts (verbal and/or behavioral) in response to common stressors, averaging at least three per week, for at least 12 months. The outbursts must occur in at least two distinct settings (e.g., home, school, or with peers), be severe in at least one setting, begin before age 10 years, and be characterized by the following <u>three</u> symptoms.

   i. Temper or behavioral outbursts: *When you get upset or lose your temper, what happens? Do you yell? Do you slap, punch, bite, or hit another person? Do you break or destroy things?*

   ii. Disproportionate reaction: *When you get upset or lose your temper, do you know what sets you off? What kinds of things bother you so much that you feel like yelling or hitting?*

   iii. Persistently irritable or angry mood between temper outbursts: *When you are not yelling or upset, how do you feel inside? Do you usually feel grouchy, angry, irritable, or sad?*

b. Exclusions

   i. These responses must be inconsistent with a child's developmental level.

ii. If the behaviors occur exclusively during an episode of major depressive disorder or are better explained by another mental disorder (e.g., autism spectrum disorder, posttraumatic stress disorder (PTSD), separation anxiety disorder, persistent depressive disorder), do not make the diagnosis.

iii. If the symptoms are attributable to the physiological effects of a substance or to another medical or neurological condition, do not make the diagnosis.

iv. If a child is currently diagnosed with oppositional defiant disorder, intermittent explosive disorder, or bipolar disorder, do not make the diagnosis.

c. Alternative: If, during the past year, there was a period lasting more than a day during which the child exhibited abnormally elevated mood and three criteria for a manic episode, consider the possibility of a bipolar disorder (see DSM-5-TR, pp. 139–175).

Anxiety Disorders

DSM-5-TR pp. 215–261

Screening questions: *Would you say that you worry a lot or more than other kids your age? Do people say that you worry too much or are too shy? Do you feel afraid when you're alone or away from your family? Do you get scared about going to school? Is it hard for you to control or stop your worrying? Are there specific things, places, or situations that make you feel very anxious or afraid? Have you ever felt suddenly frightened, nervous, or anxious for no reason at all? If so, can you tell me about that?*

If yes, ask: *Do these experiences ever cause you significant trouble with your friends or family, at school, or in another setting?*

- If a specific phobia is elicited, proceed to specific phobia criteria.
- If no, first proceed to panic disorder criteria. Then proceed to generalized anxiety disorder criteria.

1. Specific Phobia

   a. Inclusion: Requires that for at least 6 months, a person has experienced marked fear or anxiety as characterized by the following <u>three</u> symptoms.

i. Specific fear: *Do you fear a specific object or situation, such as flying, heights, animals, or something else, so much that being exposed to it makes you feel immediately afraid or anxious? What is it?*

ii. Fear or anxiety provoked by exposure: *When you encounter this, do you experience an immediate sense of fear or anxiety, cry, throw tantrums, or hold on to a parent?*

iii. Avoidance: *Do you find yourself taking steps to avoid this? What are they? When you must encounter this, do you experience intense fear or anxiety, cry, throw tantrums, or hold on to a parent?*

b. Exclusion: The fear, anxiety, and avoidance are not restricted to objects or situations related to obsessions, reminders of traumatic events, separation from home or attachment figures, or social situations.

c. Modifiers

i. Specifiers
- Descriptive
  - Animal
  - Natural environment
  - Blood-injection-injury
  - Situational
  - Other

d. Alternatives

i. If a young person reports developmentally inappropriate and excessive distress when separated from home or a major attachment figure or expresses persistent worry that their major attachment figure will be harmed or will die, which results in reluctance or refusal to be separated from home or a major attachment figure, consider separation anxiety disorder (full criteria are in DSM-5-TR, p. 217). The onset of this disorder is before age 18. The minimum duration of symptoms necessary to meet the diagnostic criteria is 4 weeks for children and adolescents.

ii. If a young person consistently fails to speak in specific social situations for at least 1 month and this interferes with educational or occupational achievement, consider selective mutism (full criteria are in DSM-5-TR, p. 222). If the disturbance is due to a lack of knowledge of, or comfort with, the spoken language, do not make the diagnosis. If the disturbance is better explained by a communication disorder, autism spectrum disorder, or psychotic disorder, do not make the diagnosis.

iii. If a young person reports at least 6 months of marked and disproportionate fear or anxiety about situations such as public transportation, open spaces, being in enclosed spaces, standing in line or being in a crowd, or being outside the home alone, and if these fears cause them to actively avoid these situations, consider agoraphobia (full criteria are in DSM-5-TR, p. 246).

iv. If a young person reports at least 6 months of marked fear or anxiety about, or avoidance of, social situations in which they fear other people will observe or scrutinize them out of proportion to the actual threat posed by these social situations, and the fear, anxiety, or avoidance causes clinically significant distress or impairment, consider social anxiety disorder (full criteria are in DSM-5-TR, pp. 229–230). In children, the anxiety must occur with peers, not just with adults. Children may express fear or anxiety by crying, throwing tantrums, freezing, clinging, shrinking, or failing to speak in social situations.

2. Panic Disorder

a. Inclusion: Requires recurrent panic attacks, as characterized by at least <u>four</u> of the following symptoms.

i. Palpitations, pounding heart, or accelerated heart rate: *When you experience these sudden surges of intense fear or discomfort, does your heart race or pound?*

ii. Sweating: *During these events, do you find yourself sweating more than usual?*

iii. Trembling or shaking: *During these events, do you shake or develop a tremor?*

iv. Sensations of shortness of breath or smothering: *During these events, do you feel like you are being smothered or cannot catch your breath?*

v. Feelings of choking: *During these events, do you feel as though you are choking, as if something is blocking your throat?*

vi. Chest pain or discomfort: *During these events, do you feel intense pain or discomfort in your chest?*

    vii. Nausea or abdominal distress: *During these events, do you feel sick to your stomach or like you need to vomit?*

   viii. Feeling dizzy, unsteady, light-headed, or faint: *During these events, do you feel dizzy, light-headed, or like you may faint?*

    ix. Chills or heat sensations: *During these events, do you feel very cold and shiver, or do you feel intensely hot?*

     x. Paresthesias: *During these events, do you feel numbness or tingling?*

    xi. Derealization or depersonalization: *During these events, do you feel like people or places that are familiar to you are unreal or that you are so detached from your body that it is like you are standing outside your body or watching yourself?*

    xii. Fear of losing control: *During these events, do you fear you may be losing control or even "going crazy"?*

   xiii. Fear of dying: *During these events, do you fear you may be dying?*

b. Inclusion: At least <u>one</u> panic attack is followed by at least 1 month of at least <u>one</u> of the following symptoms.

     i. Persistent worry about consequences: *Are you persistently concerned or worried about additional panic attacks? Are you persistently concerned or worried that these attacks mean you are having a heart attack, losing control, or "going crazy"?*

    ii. Maladaptive changes to avoid attacks: *Have you made significant changes in your behavior, such as avoiding unfamiliar situations or exercise, to avoid attacks?*

c. Exclusion: If the disturbance is better explained by another mental disorder or is attributable to the physiological effects of a substance or medication or another medical condition, do not make the diagnosis.

d. Alternatives: If a young person reports panic attacks as described above but neither experiences persistent worry about consequences nor makes maladaptive changes to avoid attacks, consider using the panic attack specifier (see DSM-5-TR, p. 242). The panic attack specifier can be used with other anxiety disorders as well as with depressive, traumatic, and substance use disorders.

3. Generalized Anxiety Disorder

    a. Inclusion: Requires excessive anxiety and worry that is difficult to control, occurring more days than not for at least 6 months, about several events or activities (such as school performance), associated with at least <u>three</u> of the following symptoms.

        i. Restlessness: *When you think about events or activities that make you anxious or worried, do you feel restless, on edge, or keyed up?*

        ii. Easily fatigued: *Do you find that you often tire or fatigue easily?*

        iii. Difficulty concentrating: *When you are anxious or worried, do you often find it hard to concentrate or find that your mind goes blank?*

        iv. Irritability: *When you are anxious or worried, do you often feel irritable or easily annoyed?*

        v. Muscle tension: *When you get anxious or worried, do you often experience muscle tightness or tension?*

        vi. Sleep disturbance: *Do you find it difficult to fall asleep or stay asleep or experience restless and unsatisfying sleep?*

    b. Exclusion: If the anxiety and worry are better explained by another mental disorder or are attributable to the physiological effects of a substance or medication or another medical condition, do not make the diagnosis.

    c. Alternatives

        i. If a substance, including a medication prescribed to treat a mental disorder, directly causes the episode, consider a substance/medication-induced anxiety disorder (full criteria are in DSM-5-TR, pp. 255–256).

        ii. If another medical condition directly causes the anxiety and worry, consider an anxiety disorder due to another medical condition (full criteria are in DSM-5-TR, pp. 258–259).

        iii. If a young person experiences symptoms characteristic of an anxiety disorder that cause clinically significant distress or functional impairment without meeting full criteria for another anxiety disorder, consider unspecified anxiety disorder (see DSM-5-TR, p. 261). If you wish to communicate the specific reason why a young person's symptoms do not meet the criteria for a specific anxiety disorder, consider other specified anxiety disorder (see DSM-5-TR, p. 261). Examples include *khyâl cap* (wind attacks), *ataque de nervios* (attack of nerves), and generalized anxiety not occurring more days than not.

Obsessive-Compulsive and Related Disorders

DSM-5-TR pp. 263–294

Screening questions: *Do you frequently experience intrusive and unwanted images, thoughts, or urges? Are there any physical acts that you feel like you must do to avoid or reduce the distress associated with these images, thoughts or urges?*

If yes, ask: *Do these experiences or behaviors ever cause you significant trouble with your friends or family, at school, or in another setting?*

- If yes, proceed to obsessive-compulsive disorder (OCD) criteria.
- If no, proceed to the body-focused repetitive behavior screening question, which follows the OCD section.

1. Obsessive-Compulsive Disorder

   a. Inclusion: Requires the presence of obsessive thoughts, compulsive behaviors, or both, as manifested by <u>all</u> of the following symptoms.

      i. Obsessive thoughts (as defined by both questions): *When you experience these intrusive and unwanted images, thoughts, or urges, do they make you really anxious or distressed? Do you have to work hard to ignore or suppress these kinds of thoughts?*

      ii. Compulsive behaviors (as defined by both questions): *Some people try to reverse intrusive ideas by repeatedly performing some kind of action such as hand washing or lock checking or by performing a mental act such as counting, praying, or silently repeating words. Do you do something like that? Do you think that doing so will reduce your distress or prevent something you dread from occurring?*

b. Inclusion: The obsessions or compulsions are time-consuming (e.g., take more than 1 hour per day) or cause clinically significant distress or impairment.

c. Exclusions

   i. If the obsessions or compulsions are better explained by another mental disorder, do not make the diagnosis. If the obsessive-compulsive symptoms are due to the physiological effects of a substance, do not make the diagnosis.

   ii. If a young person reports that their intrusive images, thoughts, or urges are pleasurable, their symptoms do not meet the criteria for OCD. Instead, consider substance use disorders, personality disorders, and paraphilic disorders.

   iii. Exclusion: If a young person reports intrusive images, thoughts, or urges centered on more real-world concerns, consider an anxiety disorder.

d. Modifiers

   i. Specifiers

      • Insight

         • With good or fair insight: Use if a young person recognizes that their beliefs are definitely or probably untrue.
         • With poor insight: Use if a young person thinks their beliefs are probably true.
         • With absent insight/delusional beliefs: Use if a young person is completely convinced their beliefs are true.

   ii. Tic-related: Use if a young person's symptoms meet criteria for a current or lifetime chronic tic disorder.

e. Alternatives

   i. If a young person reports intrusive images, thoughts, or urges centered on their body image, consider body dysmorphic disorder (full criteria are in DSM-5-TR, pp. 271–272). The criteria include preoccupation with perceived defects in physical appearance beyond concern about weight or body fat in a person with an eating disorder, repetitive behaviors or mental acts in response to concern about appearance, and clinically significant distress or impairments because of the preoccupation.

ii. If a young person reports persistent difficulty with parting with possessions regardless of their value, consider hoarding disorder (full criteria are in DSM-5-TR, p. 277). The criteria include strong urges to save items, distress associated with discarding items, and the accumulation of many possessions that clutter the home or workplace to the extent that it can no longer be used for its intended function.

iii. If a substance, including a substance prescribed to treat depression, directly causes the condition, consider substance/medication-induced obsessive-compulsive and related disorder (full criteria are in DSM-5-TR, pp. 287–289).

iv. If another medical condition directly causes the episode, consider obsessive-compulsive and related disorder due to another medical condition (full criteria are in DSM-5-TR, p. 291).

v. If a young person experiences symptoms characteristic of an obsessive-compulsive and related disorder that cause clinically significant distress or functional impairment without meeting full criteria for another obsessive-compulsive and related disorder, consider unspecified obsessive-compulsive and related disorder (see DSM-5-TR, p. 294). If you wish to communicate the specific reason why a person's symptoms do not meet the criteria for a specific obsessive-compulsive and related disorder, consider other specified obsessive-compulsive and related disorder (see DSM-5-TR, pp. 293–294). Examples include body dysmorphic–like disorder with actual flaws, body dysmorphic–like disorder without repetitive behaviors, body-focused repetitive behavior disorder, obsessional jealousy, olfactory reference disorder, *shubo-kyofu*, and *koro*.

2. Body-Focused Repetitive Behaviors

a. Inclusion: DSM-5-TR includes two conditions, trichotillomania (hair-pulling disorder) and excoriation (skin-picking) disorder, with identically structured criteria. Either diagnosis requires the presence of <u>all</u> <u>three</u> of the following symptoms.

    i. Behavior: *Do you frequently pull your hair or pick at your skin so much that it has caused hair loss or skin lesions?*

    ii. Repeated attempts to change: *Have you repeatedly tried to decrease or stop this behavior?*

    iii. Impairment: *Does this behavior cause you to feel ashamed or out of control? Do you avoid school, social settings, or work because of these behaviors?*

  b. Exclusion

    i. If the behavior is due to another medical condition, is better explained by another mental disorder, or is a result of substance use, you should not diagnose either trichotillomania or excoriation disorder.

Trauma- and Stressor-Related Disorders

DSM-5-TR pp. 295–328

Screening questions: *What is the worst thing that has ever happened to you? Has anyone ever touched you in a way you did not want? Have you ever experienced or witnessed an event in which you were seriously injured or your life was in danger or you thought you were going to be seriously injured or endangered?*

If yes, ask: *Do you think about or reexperience these events? Does thinking about these experiences ever cause significant trouble with your friends or family, at school, or in another setting?*

- If yes, proceed to PTSD criteria.
- If a child says no but their family or caregivers report disturbances in the child's primary attachments, proceed to reactive attachment disorder criteria.

1. Posttraumatic Stress Disorder

  a. Inclusion: Requires exposure to actual or threatened death, serious injury, or sexual violation in at least one of the following ways: direct experience; in-person witnessing; learning of actual or threatened death, serious injury, or sexual violation of a close family member or friend; repeated or extreme exposure to aversive details of traumatic event(s). In a child 6 years or younger, the traumatic exposure can be learning of the trauma experienced by a parent or caregiver. In addition, a person must experience at least <u>one</u> of the following intrusion symptoms for at least 1 month after the traumatic experience.

  i. Memories: *After that experience, did you ever experience intrusive memories of the experience when you did not want to think about it?* For young children, repetitive reenactment through play qualifies: *Do you repeatedly reenact that experience with your toys or dolls when playing?*
  ii. Dreams: *Did you have recurrent, distressing dreams related to the experience?* For young children, frightening dreams without recognizable content qualifies: *Do you frequently have very frightening dreams that you cannot recall or describe?*
  iii. Flashbacks: *After that experience, did you ever feel as if it were happening to you again, like in a flashback?* For young children, this may be observed in their play.
  iv. Exposure distress: *When you are around people, places, and objects that remind you of that experience, do you feel intense or prolonged distress?*
  v. Physiological reactions: *When you are around people, places, or objects that remind you of that experience, do you have distressing physical responses?*

b. Inclusion: In addition, a young person older than 6 years must experience at least <u>one</u> of the following avoidance symptoms after the traumatic experience. For a child 6 years or younger, no negative mood symptoms need be experienced if at least <u>one</u> negative mood symptom (see item (c) below) is present.

  i. Internal reminders: *Do you work hard to avoid thoughts, feelings, or physical sensations that bring up memories of this experience?*
  ii. External reminders: *Do you work hard to avoid people, places, and objects that bring up memories of this experience?*

c. Inclusion: In addition, a young person older than 6 years must experience at least <u>two</u> of the following negative symptoms. For a child 6 years or younger, no negative mood symptoms need be experienced if at least <u>one</u> avoidance symptom (see (b) above) is present.

i. Impaired memory: *Do you have trouble remembering important parts of the experience?*

ii. Negative self-image: *Do you frequently think negative thoughts about yourself, other people, or the world?*

iii. Blame: *Do you frequently blame yourself or others for your experience, even when you know that you or they were not responsible?*

iv. Negative emotional state: *Do you stay down, angry, ashamed, or fearful most of the time?*

v. Decreased participation: *Are you much less interested in activities in which you used to participate?*

vi. Detachment: *Do you feel detached or estranged from the people in your life because of this experience?*

vii. Inability to experience positive emotions: *Do you find that you cannot feel happy, loved, or satisfied? Do you feel numb, or like you cannot love?*

d. Inclusion: In addition, a young person must experience at least <u>two</u> of the following arousal behaviors.

i. Irritable or aggressive: *Do you often act very grumpy or get aggressive?*

ii. Recklessness: *Do you often act reckless or self-destructive?*

iii. Hypervigilance: *Are you always on edge or keyed up?*

iv. Exaggerated startle: *Do you startle easily?*

v. Impaired concentration: *Do you often have trouble concentrating on a task or problem?*

vi. Sleep disturbance: *Do you often have difficulty falling asleep or staying asleep, or do you often wake up without feeling rested?*

e. Exclusion: The episode is not directly caused by a substance or by another medical condition.

f. Modifiers

i. Subtypes

- With dissociative symptoms, either depersonalization or derealization

ii. Specifier

- With delayed expression: Use if a person does not exhibit all the diagnostic criteria until at least 6 months after the traumatic experience.

g. Alternatives

i. If the episode lasts less than 1 month and the experience occurred within the past month, and the young person experiences at least <u>nine</u> of the posttraumatic symptoms described above, consider acute stress disorder (full criteria are in DSM-5-TR, pp. 313–315).

ii. If the episode began within 3 months of the experience and a young person's symptoms do not meet the symptomatic and behavioral criteria for PTSD, consider an adjustment disorder (full criteria are in DSM-5-TR, pp. 319–320). The criteria include marked distress disproportionate to an acute stressor, either traumatic or nontraumatic, and significant impairment in function.

iii. If a young person experiences symptoms characteristic of a trauma- and stressor-related disorder that cause clinically significant distress or functional impairment without meeting full criteria for one of the named disorders, consider unspecified trauma- and stressor-related disorder (see DSM-5-TR, p. 328). If you wish to communicate the specific reason why a young person's symptoms do not meet the criteria for a specific disorder, consider other specified trauma- and stressor-related disorder (see DSM-5-TR, pp. 327–328). Examples include prolonged grief disorder and adjustment-like disorders with delayed onset of symptoms that occur more than 3 months after the stressor.

iv. If a young person experiences persistent grief after the death of someone they were close to, consider prolonged grief disorder (see DSM-5-TR, pp. 322–323). The death must have occurred at least 6 months ago for symptoms to meet criteria. For the criteria to be met, a person must experience, nearly daily, intense yearning or longing for the deceased or preoccupation with thoughts or memories of the deceased that exceeds expected cultural or social norms. For the criteria to be met, the person must have been experiencing <u>three</u> or more of these symptoms nearly daily for the past month: identity disruption, a marked sense of disbelief about the death, avoidance of reminders that the person is dead, intense emotional pain, difficulty reintegrating into activi-

ties and relationships, emotional numbness, a feeling that life is meaningless, and intense loneliness.

2. Reactive Attachment Disorder

This section contains questions phrased for interviewing an
older child with an ability to self-reflect. For younger children or those with limited cognitive functioning, rephrase
these questions to interview the child's caregiver instead.

- a. Inclusion: Requires that a child experience pathogenic
  care, before age 5 years, that results in both of the following behaviors.

  - i. Rare or minimal comfort seeking: *When you are
    feeling really angry, upset, or sad, do you avoid comfort
    or consolation from other people?*
  - ii. Rare or minimal response to comfort: *When you are
    feeling really angry, upset, or sad, and somebody says
    or does something nice for you, does it make you feel a
    little better?*

- b. Inclusion: Requires the persistent experience of at
  least two of the following states.

  - i. Relative lack of social and emotional responsive-
    ness to others: *When you interact with other people,
    do you usually have very little feeling or emotion?*
  - ii. Limited positive affect: *Do you usually find it hard
    to be excited or to feel good or cheerful?*
  - iii. Episodes of unexplained irritability, sadness, or
    fearfulness that are evident during nonthreaten-
    ing interactions with caregivers: *Do you often have
    episodes where you become irritable, sad, or afraid with
    an adult caregiver who does not pose a threat to you?*

- c. Inclusion: Requires the persistent experience of at
  least one of the following states that should be as-
  sessed in the social history.

  - i. Social neglect or deprivation in the form of per-
    sistent lack of having basic emotional needs for
    comfort, stimulation, and affection met
  - ii. Repeated changes of primary caregivers that limit
    opportunities to form stable attachments
  - iii. Rearing in unusual settings that severely limit op-
    portunities to form selective attachments

d. Exclusions

   i. If a child does not have a developmental age of at least 9 months, do not make the diagnosis.

   ii. If a child's symptoms meet criteria for autism spectrum disorder, do not make the diagnosis.

e. Modifiers

   i. Specifier

   - Persistent: Use when the disorder is present for more than 12 months.

   ii. Severity: Specified severe when a child has all symptoms of the disorder, with each symptom manifesting in relatively high levels.

f. Alternative: If a young child who has experienced extremes of insufficient care shows profoundly disturbed externalizing behavior, consider disinhibited social engagement disorder (full criteria are in DSM-5-TR, pp. 298–299). The criteria include at least two of the following symptoms: reduced reticence with unfamiliar adults, overly familiar verbal or physical behavior, diminished checking back with adult caregiver after venturing away, and a willingness to go off with an unfamiliar adult with reduced hesitation.

Dissociative Disorders

DSM-5-TR pp. 329–348

Screening questions: *Everyone has trouble remembering things sometimes, but do you ever lose time, forget important details about yourself, or find evidence that you took part in events that you cannot recall? Do you ever feel as if people or places that are familiar to you are unreal or that you are so detached from your body that it is like you are standing outside your body or watching yourself?*

   If yes, ask: *Did these experiences ever cause you significant trouble with your friends or family, at school, or in another setting?*

- If amnesia predominates, proceed to dissociative amnesia criteria.
- If depersonalization or derealization predominates, proceed to depersonalization/derealization disorder criteria.

1. Dissociative Amnesia

   a. Inclusion: Requires the presence of an inability to re-call important autobiographical information beyond ordinary forgetting, most often manifested by at least <u>one</u> of the following symptoms.

      i. Localized or selective amnesia: *Do you find yourself unable to recall a really important event, especially events that were especially stressful or even traumatic?*

      ii. Generalized amnesia: *Do you find yourself unable to recall really important moments in your life history or details of your very identity?*

   b. Exclusions

      i. If the disturbance is better accounted for by disso-ciative identity disorder, PTSD, acute stress disor-der, or somatic symptom disorder, do not make the diagnosis.

      ii. If the disturbance is due to the physiological ef-fects of a substance or a neurological or other medical condition, do not make the diagnosis.

   c. Modifiers

      i. Specifier

         • With dissociative fugue: Use when a person engages in purposeful travel or bewildered wandering for which they have amnesia.

   d. Alternative: If a young person reports a disruption of identity, characterized by two or more distinct personal-ity states or an experience of possession, that causes clin-ically significant distress and functional impairment, consider dissociative identity disorder (full criteria are in DSM-5-TR, p. 330). The criteria include recurrent gaps in recall that are inconsistent with ordinary forgetting and dissociative experiences that are not a normal part of a broadly accepted cultural or religious practice and that are not attributable to the physiological effects of a sub-stance or another medical condition.

2. Depersonalization/Derealization Disorder

   a. Inclusion: Requires at least <u>one</u> of the following man-ifestations.

      i. Depersonalization: *Do you frequently have experi-ences of unreality or detachment—like you are an out-*

side observer of your mind, thoughts, feelings, sensations, body, or whole self?

    ii. Derealization: *Do you frequently have experiences of unreality or detachment for your surroundings—like you often experience people or places as unreal, dream-like, foggy, lifeless, or visually distorted?*

  b. Inclusion: Requires intact reality testing. *During these experiences, can you distinguish the experiences from actual events—what is occurring outside of you?*

  c. Exclusions

    i. If the disturbance is due to the physiological effects of a substance or a neurological or other medical condition, do not make the diagnosis.

    ii. If depersonalization or derealization occurs exclusively as a symptom of or during another mental disorder, do not make the diagnosis.

  d. Alternative: If a young person is experiencing a disorder whose most prominent symptoms are amnestic but do not meet the criteria for a specific disorder, consider other specified dissociative disorder (see DSM-5-TR, pp. 347–348). Examples include subthreshold dissociative disturbances in identity and memory, chronic and recurrent syndromes of mixed dissociative symptoms, identity disturbances in individuals subjected to prolonged periods of intense coercive persuasion, acute reactions to stressful situations, acute psychotic states intermixed with dissociative symptoms in a person whose symptoms do not meet criteria for delirium or a psychotic disorder, and dissociative trance.

Somatic Symptom and Related Disorders

DSM-5-TR pp. 349–370

Screening questions: *Do you worry about your physical health more than most young people do? Do you get sick more often than most young people?*

    If yes, ask: *Do these experiences significantly affect your daily life at home or in school?*

    If yes, ask: *Which is worse for you: worrying about the symptoms you experience or worrying about your health and the possibility that you are sick?*

- If worry about symptoms predominates, proceed to somatic symptom disorder criteria.
- If worry about being ill or sick predominates, proceed to illness anxiety disorder criteria.

1. Somatic Symptom Disorder

   a. Inclusion: Requires at least <u>one</u> somatic symptom that is distressing. *Do you experience unexplained symptoms that cause you to feel anxious or distressed? Do these symptoms significantly disrupt your daily life?*

   b. Inclusion: Requires at least <u>one</u> of the following thoughts, feelings, or behaviors for at least 6 months.

      i. Disproportionate thoughts: *Do you find yourself persistently thinking about your health concerns and how serious they are?*

      ii. Persistently high level of anxiety: *Do you persistently feel a high level of anxiety or worry about your health concerns?*

      iii. Excessive investment: *Do you find yourself investing a lot more time and energy into your health concerns than you would like to?*

   c. Modifiers

      i. Specifiers
         - With predominant pain
         - Persistent

      ii. Severity
         - Mild: One of the symptoms specified in (b) above
         - Moderate: Two or more of the symptoms specified in (b) above
         - Severe: Two or more of the symptoms specified in (b) above plus multiple somatic complaints (or one very severe somatic symptom)

   d. Alternatives

      i. If a young person is focused on the loss of bodily function rather than on the distress a particular symptom causes, consider functional neurological symptom disorder (conversion disorder) (full criteria are in DSM-5-TR, pp. 360–361). The criteria for this disorder include symptoms of altered voluntary motor or sensory function, clinical evidence that these symptoms or deficits are inconsistent with recognized medical or neurological conditions, and significant impairment in social or occupational functioning. When possible, specify the symptom type using available specifiers, including with weakness or paralysis, with abnormal movement, with swallowing symptoms, with speech symptoms, with attacks or seizures, and with special sensory symptoms.

ii. If a young person has a documented medical condition other than a mental disorder, but behavioral or psychological factors adversely affect the course of their medical condition by delaying recovery, decreasing adherence, significantly increasing health risks, or influencing the underlying pathophysiology, consider psychological factors affecting other medical conditions (full criteria are in DSM-5-TR, pp. 364–365).

iii. If a young person falsifies physical or psychological signs or symptoms, or induces injury or disease to deceptively present themselves to others as ill, impaired, or injured, consider factitious disorder imposed on self (full criteria are in DSM-5-TR, p. 367). For the criteria to be met, the young person needs to exhibit these behaviors even in the absence of obvious external rewards. The symptoms cannot be better accounted for by another mental disorder, such as a psychotic disorder.

iv. If a young person falsifies physical or psychological signs or symptoms or induces injury or disease to deceptively present someone else to others as ill, impaired, or injured, consider factitious disorder imposed on another (full criteria are in DSM-5-TR, p. 367) The diagnosis is assigned to the perpetrator rather than the victim, and for the criteria to be met, the behavior needs to occur even in the absence of obvious external rewards and cannot be better explained by another mental disorder, such as a psychotic disorder.

2. Illness Anxiety Disorder

a. Inclusion: Requires all of the following symptoms for at least 6 months and the absence of somatic symptoms.

    i. Preoccupation: *Do you find yourself unable to stop thinking about having or acquiring a serious illness?*

    ii. Anxiety: *Do you feel a high level of anxiety or worry about having or acquiring a serious illness?*

    iii. Associated behaviors: *Have these worries affected your behavior? Some people find themselves frequently checking their body for signs of illness; reading about illness all the time; or avoiding persons, places, or objects to ward off illness. Do you find yourself doing any of those things or things like that?*

b. Exclusion: If a person's symptoms are better explained by another mental disorder, do not make the diagnosis.

c. Modifiers

    i. Subtypes

      • Care-seeking
      • Care-avoidant

    ii. Course

      • Transient

d. Alternatives: If a young person endorses symptoms characteristic of a somatic symptom disorder that cause clinically significant distress or impairment without meeting the full criteria for a specific disorder, consider unspecified somatic symptom and related disorder (see DSM-5-TR, p. 370). If you wish to communicate specific reasons why full criteria are not met, consider other specified somatic symptom and related disorder (see DSM-5-TR, p. 370). Examples include brief somatic symptom disorder, brief illness anxiety disorder, illness anxiety disorder without excessive health-related behaviors, and pseudocyesis.

Feeding and Eating Disorders

DSM-5-TR pp. 371–397

Screening questions: *What do you think of your appearance? Do you avoid particular foods so much that it negatively affects your health or weight?*

    If yes, ask: *When you consider yourself, is the shape or weight of your body one of the most important things about you?*

- If yes, proceed to anorexia nervosa criteria.
- If no, proceed to avoidant/restrictive food intake disorder criteria.

1. Anorexia Nervosa

   a. Inclusion: Requires the presence of all <u>three</u> of the following features.

      i. Energy restriction leading to significantly low body weight adjusted for age, developmental trajectory, physical health, and sex: *Have you limited the food you eat to achieve a low body weight? What was the least you ever weighed? What do you weigh now?*

      ii. Fear of weight gain or behavior interfering with weight gain: *Do you have an intense fear of gaining weight or becoming fat? Has there ever been a time when you were already at a low weight and still did things to interfere with gaining weight?*

      iii. Disturbance in self-perceived weight or shape: *How do you experience the weight and shape of your body? Are there particular parts of your body that you frequently evaluate or measure? How do you think having a significantly low body weight will affect your physical health?*

   b. Modifiers

      i. Subtypes

         - Restricting type: Use when a young person reports no recurrent episodes of bingeing or purging in the past 3 months.
         - Binge-eating/purging type: Use when a young person reports recurrent episodes of bingeing or purging in the past 3 months.

      ii. Specifiers

         - In partial remission
         - In full remission

      iii. Severity (based on age- and gender-matched percentiles equivalent to adult BMI)

         - Mild: BMI ≥17 kg/m^2
         - Moderate: BMI 16–16.99 kg/m^2
         - Severe: BMI 15–15.99 kg/m^2
         - Extreme: <15 kg/m^2

c. Alternatives

    i.   If a young person reports recurrent binge eating, re-current inappropriate compensatory behaviors to prevent weight gain (e.g., misuse of laxatives or other medications, self-induced vomiting, excessive exercise), and self-image unduly influenced by the shape or weight of their body, consider bulimia nervosa (full criteria are in DSM-5-TR, pp. 387–388). The diagnosis requires that binge eating and compensatory behaviors both occur, on average, at least once a week for 3 months. The diagnosis cannot be made if bingeing and compensating behaviors occur only during episodes of anorexia nervosa.

    ii. If a young person has recurrent episodes of binge eating characterized <u>both</u> by eating an amount of food that is definitely larger than most people would eat in a similar period of time under similar circumstances and by a sense of lack of control over eating during the episode, consider binge-eating disorder (full criteria are in DSM-5-TR, pp. 392–393). Binge-eating episodes are associated with at least <u>three</u> of the following: eating much more rapidly than normal; eating until feeling uncomfortably full; eating large amounts of food when not feeling physically hungry; eating alone because of feeling embarrassed by how much one is eating; and feeling disgusted with oneself, depressed, or very guilty after overeating. For the diagnosis to be made, a person must experience marked distress regarding the binge eating and binge eating must occur, on average, at least once a week for 3 months. Finally, the binge eating cannot occur exclusively during anorexia nervosa or bulimia nervosa.

2. Avoidant/Restrictive Food Intake Disorder

    a. Inclusion: Requires significant disturbance in eating or feeding as manifested by at least <u>one</u> of the following sequelae.

        i.   Significant weight loss: *Do you avoid certain foods or restrict what you eat to the extent that you have not grown at the expected rate or have experienced a significant weight loss?*

ii. Significant nutritional deficiency: *Do you avoid or restrict food to the extent that it has negatively affected your health, as in experiencing a significant nutritional deficiency?*

iii. Dependence on enteral feeding or oral supplements: *Have you avoided or restricted food to the extent that you depend on tube feedings or oral supplements to maintain nutrition?*

iv. Marked interference with psychosocial functioning: *Has avoiding or restricting food impaired your ability to participate in your usual social activities or made it hard to form or sustain relationships? Can you eat with other people or participate in social activities when food is present?*

b. Exclusions

i. If the eating disturbance is better explained by lack of available food (e.g., food insecurity), by a culturally sanctioned practice (e.g., religious fasting), or by eating practices related to a disturbance in body image, do not make the diagnosis.

ii. If the eating disturbance is due to another medical condition or is better explained by another mental disorder, do not make the diagnosis.

c. Modifiers

i. Specifier

• In remission

d. Alternatives

i. If a young person persistently eats nonnutritive nonfood substances over a period of at least 1 month, consider pica (see DSM-5-TR, pp. 371–372). The eating of nonnutritive, nonfood substances must be inappropriate to the person's developmental stage and must not be part of a culturally supported or socially normative practice.

ii. If a young person repeatedly regurgitates food over a period of at least 1 month, consider rumination disorder (full criteria are in DSM-5-TR, p. 374). For this diagnosis to be made, the regurgitation cannot occur as the result of an associated gastrointestinal or other medical condition, and the regurgitation cannot occur exclusively during anorexia nervosa, bulimia nervosa, binge-eating disorder, or avoid-ant/restrictive food intake disorder.

iii. If a young person has an atypical, mixed, or sub-threshold disturbance in their eating and feeding, or if you lack sufficient information to make a more specific diagnosis, consider other specified feeding or eating disorder (see DSM-5-TR, p. 396) or un-specified feeding or eating disorder (see DSM-5-TR, p. 397). DSM-5-TR also allows the use of these diagnoses for specific syndromes that are not for-mally included, such as atypical anorexia nervosa, night eating syndrome, and purging disorder.

Elimination Disorders

DSM-5-TR pp. 399–405

Screening question: *Have you repeatedly leaked urine or feces onto your clothing, your bed, the floor, or another inappropriate place?*

- If leaking urine, proceed to enuresis criteria.
- If leaking feces, proceed to encopresis criteria.

1. Enuresis

   a. Inclusion

      i. Inclusion: In addition to the intentional or invol-untary repeated voiding of urine into one's bed or clothes, requires the following frequency.

      ii. Occurs at least twice a week for 3 consecutive months: *Has this occurred at least twice a week? Has it also occurred for at least 3 months in a row?*

   b. Exclusions

      i. If a child is younger than 5 years, or the equivalent developmental age, do not make the diagnosis.

      ii. If the behavior is due to the physiological effects of a substance or another medical condition through a mechanism other than constipation, do not make the diagnosis.

   c. Modifiers

      i. Nocturnal only

      ii. Diurnal only: either urge incontinence (sudden

urge symptoms) or voiding postponement (conscious deferral of micturition urges)

    iii. Nocturnal and diurnal

2. Encopresis

  a. Inclusion

    i. In addition to the intentional or involuntary repeated voiding of feces into inappropriate places (e.g., clothing, the floor), requires the following frequency.

    ii. Occurs at least monthly for at least 3 consecutive months: *Has this occurred at least once a month? Has it also occurred for at least 3 months in a row?*

  b. Exclusions

    i. If a child is younger than 4 years, or the equivalent developmental age, do not make the diagnosis.

    ii. If the behavior is due to the physiological effects of a substance or another medical condition through a mechanism other than constipation, do not make the diagnosis.

  c. Modifiers

    i. With constipation and overflow incontinence

    ii. Without constipation and overflow incontinence

  d. Alternatives

    i. If a young person experiences symptoms characteristic of an elimination disorder that cause clinically significant distress or impairment without meeting the full criteria for an elimination disorder, consider unspecified elimination disorder (see DSM-5-TR, p. 405). If you wish to communicate the specific reason why full criteria are not met, consider other specified elimination disorder (see DSM-5-TR, p. 405).

Sleep-Wake Disorders

DSM-5-TR pp. 407–476

Screening questions: *Is your sleep often inadequate or of poor quality? Alternatively, do you often experience excessive sleepiness? Have you or someone else noticed any unusual behaviors* *while you sleep? Have you or someone else noticed that you stop breathing or gasp for air while sleeping?*

- If dissatisfaction with sleep quantity or quality predominates, proceed to insomnia disorder criteria.
- If excessive sleep predominates, proceed to hypersomnolence disorder criteria.
- If an irrepressible need to sleep or sudden lapses into sleep predominate, proceed to narcolepsy criteria.
- If unusual sleep behaviors (parasomnias) predominate, proceed to restless legs syndrome criteria.
- If sleep-breathing problems predominate, proceed to obstructive sleep apnea hypopnea criteria.

1. Insomnia Disorder

    a. Inclusion: Requires dissatisfaction with sleep quantity or quality, at least 3 nights per week, for at least 3 months, as manifested by at least <u>one</u> of the following symptoms.

        i. Difficulty initiating sleep: *Do you often have trouble getting to sleep without the help of a parent or someone else?*

        ii. Difficulty maintaining sleep: *If you wake up when you wanted to be asleep, do you need the help of a parent or someone else to get back to sleep?*

        iii. Early morning awakening: *Do you often wake up earlier than you intended and find yourself unable to return to sleep?*

    b. Exclusions

        i. The sleep difficulty must occur despite adequate opportunity for sleep.

        ii. If the insomnia is better explained by or occurs exclusively during another sleep-wake disorder, is attributable to the physiological effects of a substance, or is better explained by a coexisting mental disorder or medical condition, do not make the diagnosis.

    c. Modifiers

        i. Specifiers

            - With non–sleep disorder mental comorbidity, including substance use disorders

- With other medical comorbidity
- With another sleep disorder

  ii. Course

- Episodic
- Persistent
- Recurrent

d. Alternatives

  i. If a young person experiences a persistent or recurrent pattern of sleep disruption leading to excessive sleepiness, insomnia, or both, and this disruption is primarily due to an alteration of the circadian system or to a misalignment between the endogenous circadian rhythm and the sleep-wake schedule required by the person's physical environment or social or school schedule, consider a circadian rhythm sleep-wake disorder (full criteria, along with multiple subtypes, are in DSM-5-TR, pp. 443–451). The sleep disturbance must cause clinically significant distress or functional impairment.

  ii. If substance use, intoxication, or withdrawal is etiologically related to insomnia, consider substance/medication-induced sleep disorder, insomnia type (full criteria, along with multiple subtypes, are in DSM-5-TR, pp. 468–469). The disturbance cannot be better accounted for by delirium, a non-substance-induced sleep disorder, or the sleep symptoms usually associated with an intoxication or withdrawal syndrome.

  iii. If a young person experiences symptoms characteristic of an insomnia disorder that cause clinically significant distress or impairment but the duration has been less than 3 months, consider unspecified insomnia disorder (see DSM-5-TR, p. 475). The diagnosis is reserved for insomnia symptoms that produce significant distress or functional impairment. If you wish to communicate the reason why a person's symptoms do not meet the full criteria for a specific sleep disorder, consider other specified insomnia disorder (see DSM-5-TR, p. 475).

2. Hypersomnolence Disorder

a. Inclusion: Requires excessive sleepiness at least three times per week for at least 3 months, despite a main

sleep period lasting at least 7 hours, that causes significant distress or functional impairment. The hypersomnolence is manifested by at least <u>one</u> of the following
symptoms.

    i. Recurrent periods of sleep: *Do you often have sev-
eral periods of sleep within the same day?*

    ii. Prolonged nonrestorative sleep episode: *Do you of-
ten have a main sleep episode, lasting at least 9 hours,
that is not refreshing or restorative?*

    iii. Sleep inertia: *Do you often have difficulty being fully
awake? After awakening, do you often feel groggy or
notice that you have trouble engaging in tasks or activities that would otherwise be simple for you?*

b. Exclusion: If the hypersomnia occurs exclusively
during another sleep disorder, is better accounted for
by another sleep disorder, or is attributable to the
physiological effects of a substance, do not make the
diagnosis.

c. Modifiers

    i. Specifiers

- With mental disorder, including substance use
  disorders
- With medical condition
- With another sleep disorder

    ii. Course

- Acute: Use when duration is less than 1 month.
- Subacute: Use when duration is 1–3 months.
- Persistent: Use when duration is greater than
  3 months.

    iii. Severity

- Mild: Difficulty maintaining daytime alertness
  1–2 days/week
- Moderate: Difficulty maintaining daytime
  alertness 3–4 days/week
- Severe: Difficulty maintaining daytime alertness 5–7 days/week

d. Alternative: If substance use, intoxication, or withdrawal is etiologically related to daytime sleepiness,
consider substance/medication-induced sleep disorder, daytime sleepiness type (full criteria, along with

multiple subtypes, are in DSM-5-TR, pp. 468–469). If the disturbance is better accounted for by delirium, a non-substance-induced sleep disorder, or the sleep symptoms usually associated with an intoxication or withdrawal syndrome, this diagnosis should not be used.

3. Narcolepsy

   a. Inclusion: Requires periods of an irrepressible need to sleep or lapsing into sleep, at least three times per week over the past 3 months, along with at least <u>one</u> of the following.

      i. Episodes of cataplexy: *At least a few times a month, do you find that suddenly you grimace, open your mouth wide and thrust out your tongue, or lose muscle tone throughout your body, without any obvious emotional trigger?*

      ii. Hypocretin deficiency: Measured using cerebrospinal fluid hypocretin-1 (CSF-1) immunoreactivity values.

      iii. Nocturnal sleep polysomnography showing rapid eye movement (REM) sleep latency <15 minutes or a multiple sleep latency test showing mean sleep latency <8 minutes and >2 sleep-onset REM periods.

   b. Modifiers

      i. Specifiers

         • Narcolepsy with cataplexy or hypocretin deficiency
         • Narcolepsy without cataplexy and either without hypocretin deficiency or hypocretin unmeasured
         • Narcolepsy with cataplexy or hypocretin deficiency due to a medical condition
         • Narcolepsy without cataplexy and without hypocretin deficiency due to a medical condition

      ii. Severity

         • Mild: Need for naps only once or twice per day. Sleep disturbance, if present, is mild. Cataplexy, when present, occurs less than once per week.

- Moderate: Need for multiple naps daily. Sleep may be moderately disturbed. Cataplexy, when present, occurs daily or every few days.
- Severe: Nearly constant sleepiness. Often highly disturbed nocturnal sleep (i.e., excessive movements, vivid dreaming). Cataplexy, when present, is medication-resistant, with multiple attacks daily.

4. Obstructive Sleep Apnea Hypopnea

a. Inclusion: Requires repeated episodes of upper airway obstruction during sleep. There must be polysomnographic evidence of at least five obstructive apneas or hypopneas per hour of sleep and <u>either</u> of the following symptoms.

   i. Nocturnal breathing disturbances: *Do you often disturb your parents, siblings, or anyone else with snoring, snorting, gasping for air, or breathing pauses during sleep?*

   ii. Daytime sleepiness, fatigue, or nonrestorative sleep: *When you have an opportunity to get sleep, do you still wake up the next day feeling exhausted, sleepy, or fatigued?*

b. Inclusion: Alternatively, the diagnosis can be made by polysomnographic evidence of 15 or more obstructive apneas or hypopneas per hour of sleep regardless of accompanying symptoms.

c. Modifiers

   i. Severity

      - Mild: Use when a young person's apnea hypopnea index is less than 15.
      - Moderate: Use when a young person's apnea hypopnea index is between 15 and 30.
      - Severe: Use when a young person's apnea hypopnea index is greater than 30.

d. Alternatives

   i. If a young person demonstrates five or more central apneas per hour of sleep during polysomnographic examination, and this disturbance is not better accounted for by another current sleep disorder, consider central sleep apnea (full criteria are in DSM-5-TR, pp. 435–436).

ii. If a young person demonstrates episodes of shallow breathing associated with arterial oxygen desaturation and/or elevated carbon dioxide levels during polysomnographic examination, and this disturbance is not better accounted for by another current sleep disorder, consider sleep-related hypoventilation (full criteria are in DSM-5-TR, pp. 439–440). This disorder is most commonly associated with medical or neurological disorders, obesity, medication use, or substance use disorders.

5. Restless Legs Syndrome

a. Inclusion: Requires an urge to move the legs, usually accompanied by or in response to uncomfortable and unpleasant sensations in the legs, at least three times per week for at least 3 months, as manifested by <u>all</u> of the following symptoms.

i. Urge to move legs: *While you are asleep, do you often experience uncomfortable or unpleasant sensations in the legs? Do you often experience an urge to move your legs when you are otherwise inactive?*

ii. Relieved with movement: *Are these symptoms partially or completely relieved by moving your legs?*

iii. Nocturnal worsening: *At what times of day do you most experience the urge to move your legs? Is it worse in the evening or at night, no matter what you have done during the day?*

b. Exclusion: If a young person's symptoms are better explained by another mental disorder, another medical condition, or a behavioral condition, do not make the diagnosis.

c. Alternatives

i. If a young person experiences recurrent episodes of incomplete awakening from sleep in which they experience an abrupt and terrifying awakening (sleep terror) or they rise from bed and walk about (sleepwalking), usually during the first third of the major sleep episode, consider non–rapid eye movement sleep arousal disorders (full criteria are in DSM-5-TR, p. 452). When experiencing an episode, the person experiences little to no dream imagery. The person experiences amnesia for the episode and is relatively unresponsive to efforts of other people to communicate with them, wake them, or comfort them.

ii. If a young person repeatedly experiences extremely dysphoric and well-remembered dreams and rapidly becomes alert and oriented on awakening from these dysphoric dreams, consider nightmare disorder (full criteria are in DSM-5-TR, p. 457). The dream disturbance, or the sleep disturbance produced by awakening from the nightmare, causes clinically significant distress or functional impairment. The dysphoric dreams do not occur exclusively during another mental disorder or are not a physiological effect of a substance or medication or another medical condition.

iii. If a young person repeatedly experiences episodes of arousal from sleep associated with vocalization and/or complex motor behaviors sufficient to result in injury to themselves or their bed partner, consider rapid eye movement sleep behavior disorder (full criteria are in DSM-5-TR, p. 461). These behaviors arise during REM sleep and typically occur more than 90 minutes after sleep onset. On awakening, the person is fully awake, alert, and oriented. The diagnosis requires <u>either</u> polysomnographic evidence of REM sleep disturbance or evidence that the behaviors are injurious, potentially injurious, or disruptive.

iv. If substance or medication use, intoxication, or withdrawal is etiologically related to a parasomnia, consider substance/medication-induced sleep disorder, parasomnia type (full criteria are in DSM-5-TR, pp. 468–469). The disturbance cannot be better accounted for by delirium, a non-substance-induced sleep disorder, or the sleep symptoms usually associated with an intoxication or withdrawal syndrome. The disorder must cause significant distress or functional impairment.

v. If a young person has an atypical, mixed, or subthreshold disturbance in sleeping and waking, consider other specified sleep-wake disorder or unspecified sleep-wake disorder (see DSM-5-TR, p. 476).

Gender Dysphoria

DSM-5-TR pp. 511–520

Screening question: *Are you really uncomfortable with your assigned gender?*

If yes, ask: *Has this discomfort lasted at least 6 months and gotten to the point where you really feel that your assigned gender is incongruent with your gender identity? Does this discomfort cause significant trouble with your friends or family, at school, or in another setting?*

- If a child says yes, proceed to gender dysphoria in children.
- If an adolescent says yes, proceed to gender dysphoria in adolescents.

1. Gender Dysphoria in Children

   a. Inclusion: Requires at least <u>six</u> of the following manifestations (one of which must be a strong desire to be of the other gender) for at least 6 months' duration.

      i. Desire to be of the other gender: *Have you experienced a strong desire to be of a gender other than your assigned gender? Do you insist that people treat you as a member of a gender other than your assigned gender?*

      ii. Cross-dressing: *Do you have a strong preference for clothes usually associated with a gender other than your assigned gender?*

      iii. Cross-gender fantasy: *When you play fantasy games, do you have a strong preference for cross-gender roles?*

      iv. Cross-gender play: *When you play, do you have a strong preference for toys or activities that most people associate with the other gender?*

      v. Cross-gender playmates: *Do you have a strong preference for friends of the other gender?*

      vi. Rejection of toys, games, and activities: *Do you strongly reject the toys, games, and activities typically associated with your assigned gender?*

      vii. Dislike of anatomy: *Do you have a strong dislike for your sexual anatomy?*

      viii. Desire to have other sex characteristics: *Have you experienced a strong desire for the primary or second-*

ary sex characteristics that match your experience of gender?*

   b. Specifier

- With a disorder/difference of sex development

2. Gender Dysphoria in Adolescents

   a. Inclusion: Requires at least <u>two</u> of the following manifestations for at least 6 months' duration.

      i. Incongruence: *Have you experienced a profound sense that your primary or secondary sex characteristics do not match your gender identity?*

     ii. Desire to change: *Have you experienced a profound desire to change your primary or secondary sex characteristics because they do not match your gender identity?*

    iii. Desire to have sexual characteristics of the other gender: *Have you experienced a strong desire for the primary or secondary sex characteristics that match your experience of gender?*

    iv. Desire to be of the other gender: *Have you experienced a strong desire to be of a gender other than your assigned gender?*

     v. Desire to be treated as the other gender: *Have you experienced a strong desire to be treated as a gender other than your assigned gender?*

    vi. Conviction that one has feelings of the other gender: *Have you experienced a strong conviction that your typical feelings and reactions are those of the gender other than your assigned gender?*

   b. Modifiers

      i. Specifiers

- With a disorder/difference of sex development
- Posttransition: The individual has transitioned to full-time living in the experienced gender (with or without legalization of gender change) and has undergone (or is preparing to have) at least one gender-affirming medical procedure or treatment regimen.

   c. Alternatives

      i. If a young person experiences symptoms characteristic of gender dysphoria that cause clinically significant distress or impairment without meeting the full criteria for gender dysphoria, consider unspecified gender dysphoria (see DSM-5-TR, p. 520). If you wish to communicate the specific reason why a person's symptoms do not meet full criteria for gender dysphoria, consider other specified gender dysphoria (see DSM-5-TR, p. 520).

Disruptive, Impulse-Control, and Conduct Disorders

DSM-5-TR pp. 521–541

Screening questions: *Do you often become so upset that you make or even act on verbal threats to hurt other people, animals, or property? Have you ever been aggressive to people or animals, destroyed property, tricked other people, or stolen things?*

If yes, ask: *Have these behaviors ever caused you significant trouble with your friends or family, at school or work, with the authorities, or in another setting?*

- If persistent anger or argumentativeness predominates, proceed to oppositional defiant disorder criteria.
- If recurrent behavioral outbursts predominate, proceed to intermittent explosive disorder criteria.
- If recurrent rule breaking predominates, proceed to conduct disorder criteria.

1. Oppositional Defiant Disorder

This section contains questions phrased for interviewing an older child with an ability to self-reflect. For younger children or those with limited cognitive functioning, rephrase these questions to interview the child's caregiver instead.

    a. Inclusion: Requires a pattern of at least <u>four</u> of the following angry, argumentative, or vindictive behaviors with non-siblings over the course of more than 6 months.

    Angry/irritable mood

      i. Often loses temper: *Do you often get explosively mad at people? Does your getting really mad cause you more problems?*

      ii. Often touchy or easily annoyed: *Do you get annoyed really easily by other people?*

iii. Often angry and resentful: *Do you feel angry much of the time? Do you often feel people are making your life difficult?*

Argumentative/defiant behavior

i. Often argues with adults: *Do you often get in arguments with your parents or teachers?*

ii. Often actively defies rules or requests from authorities: *Do you often push back against rules or expectations?*

iii. Often deliberately annoys others: *Do you often push other people's buttons just to get them to react?*

iv. Often blames others for own mistakes or misbehaviors: *When you get caught doing something you aren't supposed to, are you likely to say it was someone else's fault?*

Vindictiveness

i. Has been spiteful or vindictive twice or more in past 6 months: *Have you planned to get back at people you think have wronged you and then acted on that plan?*

b. Inclusion: Behavior disturbance causes distress in the individual or others in their immediate social context or impacts functioning.

c. Exclusion: Problem does not exclusively occur from psychosis, substance abuse, depression, bipolar disorder, or disruptive mood dysregulation disorder.

d. Modifiers

i. Current severity

- Mild: symptoms in only one setting
- Moderate: symptoms in two settings
- Severe: symptoms in three or more settings

2. Intermittent Explosive Disorder

a. Inclusion: Requires recurrent behavioral outbursts in which a young person does not control aggressive impulses as manifested by <u>either</u> of the following.

i. Verbal or physical aggression: *Over the past 3 months, have you had impulsive outbursts in which you were verbally or physically aggressive toward other people, animals, or property? Have these outbursts occurred, on average, at least twice weekly?*

ii. Three behavioral outbursts involving damage to or destruction of property and/or physical assault: *Over the past 12 months, have you lost control of your behavior three or more times and destroyed property or assaulted other people?*

b. Inclusion: Also requires all <u>three</u> of the following.

i. Magnitude of aggressiveness is disproportionate to any provocation or psychosocial stressor: *Looking back at these outbursts, can you identify any events or stressors that you associate with them? Was your response much more aggressive or extreme than these events or stressors?*

ii. Recurrent outbursts are neither premeditated nor in pursuit of a tangible objective: *When you had these outbursts, did they happen when you were feeling angry or impulsive? Did the outburst occur without a clear goal, such as obtaining money or intimidating someone?*

iii. Outbursts cause marked personal distress, impair function, or are associated with financial or legal consequences: *How do these outbursts affect how you feel about yourself and how you get along with friends, family, and other people in your life? Have you ever experienced financial or legal consequences because of your outbursts?*

c. Exclusions

i. If a young person's chronological age, or equivalent developmental age, is younger than 6 years, do not make the diagnosis.

ii. If the recurrent aggressive outbursts are fully explained by another mental disorder or are attributable to another medical condition or to the physiological effects of a substance or medication, do not make the diagnosis.

iii. If aggressive behavior occurs only in the context of an adjustment disorder, do not make the diagnosis.

3. Conduct Disorder

a. Inclusion: Requires a repetitive and persistent pattern of behavior in which the basic rights of others or major age-appropriate societal norms or rules are violated, as manifested by the presence of at least <u>three</u> of the following in the past 12 months and at least <u>one</u> of the following in the past 6 months.

   i. Often bullies, threatens, or intimidates others: *Do you often bully, threaten, or intimidate other people?*

   ii. Often initiates physical fights: *Do you often start physical fights?*

  iii. Has used a weapon that can cause serious physical harm to others: *Have you used a weapon that could cause serious harm to someone else, such as a bat, brick, broken bottle, knife, or gun?*

  iv. Has been physically cruel to people: *Have you caused physical pain or suffering to other people?*

   v. Has been physically cruel to animals: *Have you caused physical pain or suffering to animals?*

  vi. Has stolen while confronting a victim: *Have you forcibly taken or stolen something from someone while the person was present?*

  vii. Has forced someone into sexual activity: *Have you forced someone into sexual activity?*

 viii. Has deliberately engaged in fire setting with the intention of causing serious damage: *Have you set fires to cause serious damage to a person, animal, or property?*

  ix. Has deliberated destroyed others' property: *Have you deliberately destroyed someone else's belongings?*

   x. Has broken into someone else's house, building, or car: *Have you broken into someone else's house, building, or car?*

  xi. Often lies to obtain goods or favors or to avoid obligations: *Do you often lie to get out of school or work or to get things you want?*

  xii. Has stolen items of nontrivial value without confronting a victim: *Have you taken or stolen something valuable from someone when the person was not present?*

 xiii. Often stays out at night despite parental prohibitions, beginning before age 13: *Before age 13, did you have a curfew, a time after which you had to be at home, that you often violated by staying out later than you were supposed to?*

 xiv. Has run away from home overnight at least twice while living in parental or parental surrogate home (or once without returning for a lengthy period): *Have you ever run away from home? How many times? Have you ever run away from home without returning for a long time?*

    xv. Is often truant from school, beginning before age 13: *Before age 13, did you often cut class or skip school?*

  b. Modifiers

    i. Subtypes

- Childhood-onset type: Use when at least one criterion symptom begins before age 10 years.
- Adolescent-onset type: Use when no criteria symptoms are present before age 10 years.
- Unspecified onset: Use when the age at onset is unknown.

    ii. Specifier

- With limited prosocial emotions: Use for a young person who persistently has at least <u>two</u> of the following characteristics: lack of remorse or guilt, callous lack of empathy, lack of concern about performance, and shallow or deficient affect. To meet criteria, these characteristics must be seen in multiple relationships and settings over at least 12 months. These characteristics reflect a person's typical pattern of interpersonal and emotional functioning and not just occasional occurrences in some situations.

    iii. Severity

- Mild: Few, if any, conduct problems beyond those required for diagnosis and relatively minor harm to others
- Moderate: Intermediate number of conduct problems and intermediate harm to others
- Severe: Many conduct problems beyond those required for diagnosis or considerable harm to others

  c. Alternatives

    i. If a young person reports deliberate and purposeful fire setting on at least two occasions, consider pyromania (full criteria are in DSM-5-TR, p. 537). The diagnosis requires tension or affective arousal before the fire setting, fascination with fire, and pleasure or relief when setting or witnessing fires. If the fire setting is done for monetary gain, to conceal criminal activity, out of anger, or in response to a hallucination, do not make the diagnosis. If the fire setting is better explained by intellectual disability, conduct disorder, mania, or antisocial personality disorder, do not make the diagnosis.

ii. If a young person repeatedly fails to resist impulses to steal objects that are not needed for the individual's personal use or their monetary value, consider kleptomania (full criteria are in DSM-5-TR, p. 539). The diagnosis requires tension or affective arousal before the theft and pleasure or relief at the time of the theft. If the stealing is done out of anger or vengeance or in response to a hallucination, do not make the diagnosis. If the stealing is better explained by conduct disorder, mania, or antisocial personality disorder, do not make the diagnosis.

iii. If a young person has symptoms characteristic of a disruptive, impulse-control, and conduct disorder that cause clinically significant distress or impairment without meeting the full criteria for a diagnosis named earlier in this section, consider unspecified disruptive, impulse-control, and conduct disorder (see DSM-5-TR, p. 541). If you wish to communicate the specific reason why a young person's symptoms do not meet the full criteria for a disruptive, impulse-control, and conduct disorder, consider other specified disruptive, impulse-control, and conduct disorder (see DSM-5-TR, p. 541).

Substance-Related and Addictive Disorders

DSM-5-TR pp. 543–665

Screening questions: *In the past year, have you drunk alcohol, smoked marijuana, or used anything else to get high? Have you ever ridden in a car with someone who was high or drinking alcohol? Do you ever use alcohol or drugs when you are alone? Do you ever use alcohol or drugs to relax?* (Knight et al. 2002)

If yes, ask: *Did these experiences ever cause you significant trouble with your friends or family, at school, or in another setting?*

- If a young person reports problems with substance use, proceed to the substance use disorder criteria for each particular substance.
- If a young person presents with substance intoxication, proceed to the substance intoxication criteria for each particular substance.
- If a young person reports problems with substance withdrawal, proceed to the substance withdrawal criteria for each particular substance.
- If a young person reports problems with gambling, proceed to gambling disorder criteria.

1. Alcohol Use Disorder

   a. Inclusion: Requires a problematic pattern of alcohol use leading to clinically significant impairment or distress as manifested by at least <u>two</u> of the following symptoms in a 12-month period.

      i. Drinking more alcohol over a longer period than intended: *When you drink, do you find that you drink more, and for a longer time, than you planned to?*

      ii. Persistent desire or unsuccessful effort to reduce alcohol use: *Do you want to cut back or stop drinking? Have you ever tried and failed to cut back or stop drinking?*

      iii. Great deal of time spent: *Do you spend a great deal of your time obtaining alcohol, drinking alcohol, or recovering from your alcohol use?*

      iv. Cravings: *Do you experience strong desires or cravings to drink alcohol?*

      v. Failure to fulfill major role obligations: *Have you repeatedly failed to fulfill major obligations at home, school, or work because of your alcohol use?*

      vi. Continued use despite awareness of interpersonal or social problems: *Do you drink alcohol even though you suspect, or even know, that it creates or worsens interpersonal or social problems?*

      vii. Giving up activities for alcohol: *Are there important social, occupational, or recreational activities that you have given up or reduced because of your alcohol use?*

viii. Use in hazardous situations: *Have you repeatedly used alcohol in situations in which it was physically hazardous, such as driving a car or operating a machine while intoxicated?*

ix. Continued use despite awareness of physical or psychological problems: *Do you drink alcohol even though you suspect, or even know, that it creates or worsens problems with your mind and body?*

x. Tolerance as manifested by <u>either</u> of the following.

- Markedly increased amounts: *Do you find that to get intoxicated or achieve the desired effect of drinking you need to consume much more alcohol than you used to?*
- Markedly diminished effects: *If you drink the same amount of alcohol as you used to, do you find that it has a lot less effect on you than it used to?*

xi. Withdrawal as manifested by <u>either</u> of the following.

- Characteristic alcohol withdrawal syndrome: *When you stop drinking, do you undergo withdrawal?*
- The same or a closely related substance is taken to relieve or avoid withdrawal symptoms: *Have you ever drunk alcohol or taken another substance to prevent alcohol withdrawal?*

b. Modifiers

i. Specifiers

- In early remission
- In sustained remission
- In a controlled environment

ii. Severity

- Mild: Use when two or three criteria are present.
- Moderate: Use when four or five criteria are present.
- Severe: Use when six or more criteria are present.

c. Alternatives

i. If a young person received more than minimal exposure to alcohol at any time during gestation and experiences neurocognitive impairment, impaired self-regulation, and deficits in adaptive functioning, consider neurodevelopmental disorder associated with prenatal alcohol exposure (see DSM-5-TR, p. 99). The diagnosis requires onset of symptoms before age 18 years and clinically significant distress or functional impairment.

    ii. If a young person experiences problems associated with the use of alcohol that are not classifiable as alcohol use disorder, intoxication, withdrawal, intoxication delirium, withdrawal delirium, alcohol-induced neurocognitive disorder, alcohol-induced psychotic disorder, alcohol-induced bipolar disorder, alcohol-induced depressive disorder, alcohol-induced anxiety disorder, alcohol-induced sexual dysfunction, or alcohol-induced sleep disorder, consider unspecified alcohol-related disorder (see DSM-5-TR, p. 568).

2. Alcohol Intoxication

    a. Inclusion: Requires at least <u>one</u> of the following signs or symptoms developing during, or shortly after, alcohol use.

        i. Slurred speech
        ii. Incoordination
        iii. Unsteady gait
        iv. Nystagmus
        v. Impairment in attention or memory
        vi. Stupor or coma

    b. Inclusion: Requires clinically significant problematic behavioral or psychological changes. *Since you began this episode of drinking, have you observed any significant changes in your behavior, mood, or judgment? Have you engaged in problematic activities, or thought problematic thoughts, that you would not have if you were sober?*

    c. Exclusion: If the symptoms are attributable to another medical condition or are better explained by another mental disorder, including intoxication with another substance, do not make the diagnosis.

3. Alcohol Withdrawal

    a. Inclusion: Requires at least <u>two</u> of the following symptoms developing within several hours to a few days of ceasing (or reducing) alcohol use that has been heavy and prolonged.

     i. Autonomic hyperactivity

    ii. Increased hand tremor

   iii. Insomnia: *Over the past couple of days, have you found it more difficult than usual to get to sleep and to stay asleep?*

   iv. Nausea or vomiting: *Over the past couple of days, have you felt sick to your stomach, felt nauseated, or even vomited?*

    v. Transient visual, tactile, or auditory hallucinations or illusions: *Over the past couple of days, have you had any experiences where you worried that your mind was playing tricks on you, such as seeing, hearing, or feeling things that other people could not?*

   vi. Psychomotor agitation

  vii. Anxiety: *Over the past couple of days, have you felt more worried or anxious than usual?*

 viii. Generalized tonic-clonic seizures

  b. Exclusion: If the symptoms are attributable to another medical condition or are better explained by another mental disorder, including intoxication with or withdrawal from another substance, do not make the diagnosis.

  c. Modifiers

    i. Specifier

      • With perceptual disturbances: Use when hallucinations occur with intact reality testing or when auditory, visual, or tactile illusions occur in the absence of delirium.

4. Caffeine Intoxication

  a. Inclusion: Requires clinically significant problematic behavioral or psychological changes shortly after ingesting caffeine, usually more than 250 mg (e.g., 2–3 cups of brewed coffee), as manifested by at least <u>five</u> of the following signs or symptoms.

    i. Restlessness: *Over the past several hours, have you felt less able to remain at rest than usual?*

   ii. Nervousness: *Over the past several hours, have you felt more jittery or nervous than usual?*

  iii. Excitement: *Over the past several hours, have you felt more excited than usual?*

  iv. Insomnia: *Over the past several hours, if you tried to sleep, did you find it more difficult than usual to get to sleep or stay asleep?*

    v. Flushed face

    vi. Diuresis: *Over the past several hours, have you urinated more often or a greater amount than usual?*

    vii. Gastrointestinal disturbance: *Over the past several hours, have you experienced an upset stomach, nausea, vomiting, or diarrhea?*

    viii. Muscle twitching: *Over the past several hours, have you noticed your muscles twitching more than usual?*

    ix. Rambling flow of thought and speech: *Over the past several hours, have you or anyone else noticed that your thoughts or speech have been long winded or even confused?*

    x. Tachycardia or cardiac arrhythmia

    xi. Periods of inexhaustibility: *Over the past several hours, have you felt as if you had so much energy it could not be used up?*

    xii. Psychomotor agitation

  b. Exclusion: If the symptoms are attributable to another medical condition or are better explained by another mental disorder, including intoxication with another substance, do not make the diagnosis.

  c. Alternative: If a young person experiences problems associated with the use of caffeine that are not classifiable as caffeine intoxication, caffeine withdrawal, caffeine-induced anxiety disorder, or caffeine-induced sleep disorder, consider unspecified caffeine-related disorder (see DSM-5-TR, p. 574).

5. Caffeine Withdrawal

  a. Inclusion: Requires at least <u>three</u> of the following symptoms developing within 24 hours of ceasing (or reducing) caffeine use that has been prolonged.

    i. Headache: *Over the past day, have you had any headaches?*

    ii. Marked fatigue or drowsiness: *Over the past day, have you felt extremely tired or sleepy?*

    iii. Dysphoric or depressed mood or irritability: *Over the past day, have you felt more down, more depressed, or even more irritable than usual?*

    iv. Difficulty concentrating: *Over the past day, have you had difficulty staying focused on a task or an activity?*

v. Flu-like symptoms: *Over the past day, have you experienced flu-like symptoms, nausea, vomiting, or muscle pain or stiffness?*

b. Exclusion: If the symptoms are attributable to another medical condition or are better explained by another mental disorder, including intoxication with or withdrawal from another substance, do not make the diagnosis.

6. Cannabis Use Disorder

a. Inclusion: Requires a problematic pattern of cannabis use leading to clinically significant impairment or distress as manifested by at least <u>two</u> of the following in a 12-month period.

i. Consuming more cannabis over a longer period than intended: *When you use cannabis, do you find that you use more, and for a longer time, than you planned to?*

ii. Persistent desire or unsuccessful effort to reduce cannabis use: *Do you want to cut back or stop using cannabis? Have you ever tried and failed to cut back or stop?*

iii. Great deal of time spent: *Do you spend a great deal of your time obtaining cannabis, using cannabis, or recovering from your cannabis use?*

iv. Cravings: *Do you experience strong desires or cravings to use cannabis?*

v. Failure to fulfill major role obligations: *Have you repeatedly failed to fulfill major obligations at home, school, or work because of your cannabis use?*

vi. Continued use despite awareness of interpersonal or social problems: *Do you use cannabis even though you suspect, or even know, that it creates or worsens interpersonal or social problems?*

vii. Giving up activities for cannabis: *Are there important social, occupational, or recreational activities that you have given up or reduced because of your cannabis use?*

viii. Use in hazardous situations: *Have you repeatedly used cannabis in situations in which it was physically hazardous, such as driving a car or operating a machine while intoxicated?*

ix. Continued use despite awareness of physical or psychological problems: *Do you use cannabis even though you suspect, or even know, that it creates or worsens problems with your mind and body?*

    x. Tolerance as manifested by <u>either</u> of the following.

- Markedly increased amounts: *Do you find that to get high or achieve the desired effect of using cannabis you need to smoke or ingest much more cannabis than you used to?*
- Markedly diminished effects: *If you use the same amount of cannabis as you used to, do you find that it has a lot less effect on you than it used to?*

    xi. Withdrawal as manifested by <u>either</u> of the following.

- Characteristic cannabis withdrawal syndrome: *When you stop using cannabis, do you undergo withdrawal?*
- The same or a related substance is taken to relieve or avoid withdrawal symptoms: *Have you used cannabis or another substance to prevent yourself from withdrawing from cannabis?*

b. Modifiers

    i. Specifiers

- In early remission
- In sustained remission
- In a controlled environment

    ii. Severity

- Mild: Use when two or three criteria are present.
- Moderate: Use when four or five criteria are present.
- Severe: Use when six or more criteria are present.

c. Alternative: If a young person experiences problems associated with the use of cannabis that are not classifiable as cannabis use disorder, intoxication, withdrawal, intoxication delirium, withdrawal delirium, cannabis-induced neurocognitive disorder, cannabis-induced psychotic disorder, cannabis-induced bipolar disorder, cannabis-induced depressive disorder, cannabis-induced anxiety disorder, cannabis-induced sexual dysfunction, or cannabis-induced sleep disorder, consider unspecified cannabis-related disorder (see DSM-5-TR, p. 586).

7. Cannabis Intoxication

a. Inclusion: Requires at least <u>two</u> of the following signs or symptoms shortly after cannabis use.

     i. Conjunctival injection

     ii. Increased appetite: *Over the past several hours, have you been much hungrier than usual?*

     iii. Dry mouth: *Over the past several hours, have you noticed that your mouth has been dry?*

     iv. Tachycardia

b. Inclusion: Requires clinically significant problematic behavioral or psychological changes. *Since you began this episode of cannabis use, have you observed any significant changes in your mood, judgment, ability to interact with others, or sense of time? Have you engaged in problematic activities, or thought problematic thoughts, that you would not have without cannabis?*

c. Exclusion: If the symptoms are attributable to another medical condition or are better explained by another mental disorder, including intoxication with another substance, do not make the diagnosis.

d. Modifiers

     i. Specifier

        • With perceptual disturbance: Use when hallucinations occur with intact reality testing or when auditory, visual, or tactile illusions occur in the absence of delirium.

8. Cannabis Withdrawal

a. Inclusion: Requires at least <u>three</u> of the following symptoms developing within 1 week of ceasing (or reducing) cannabis use that has been heavy and prolonged.

     i. Irritability, anger, or aggression: *Over the past week or so, have you felt more irritable or angry or that you were ready to confront or attack someone?*

     ii. Nervousness or anxiety: *Over the past week or so, have you felt more worried or anxious than usual?*

     iii. Sleep difficulty: *Over the past week or so, have you had any disturbing dreams or found it more difficult than usual to get to sleep and to stay asleep?*

     iv. Decreased appetite or weight loss: *Over the past week or so, have you been less hungry or even lost weight?*

     v. Restlessness: *Over the past week or so, have you felt less able to remain at rest than usual?*

vi. Depressed mood: *Over the past week or so, have you felt more down or depressed than usual?*

vii. Somatic symptoms: *Over the past week or so, have you felt any unusual physical discomfort, such as stomach pain, tremors, sweating, fever, chills, or headaches?*

b. Exclusion: If the symptoms are attributable to another medical condition or are better explained by another mental disorder, including intoxication with or withdrawal from another substance, do not make the diagnosis.

9. Phencyclidine Use Disorder or Other Hallucinogen Use Disorder

a. Inclusion: Requires a problematic pattern of phencyclidine or other hallucinogen use leading to clinically significant impairment or distress as manifested by at least <u>two</u> of the following in a 12-month period.

i. Using more phencyclidine or other hallucinogens over a longer period than intended: *When you use hallucinogens, do you find that you use more, and for a longer time, than you planned to?*

ii. Persistent desire or unsuccessful effort to reduce hallucinogen use: *Do you want to cut back or stop using hallucinogens? Have you ever tried and failed to cut back or stop using hallucinogens?*

iii. Great deal of time spent: *Do you spend a great deal of your time obtaining hallucinogens, using hallucinogens, or recovering from your hallucinogen use?*

iv. Cravings: *Do you experience strong desires or cravings to use hallucinogens?*

v. Failure to fulfill major role obligations: *Have you repeatedly failed to fulfill major obligations at home, school, or work because of your hallucinogen use?*

vi. Continued use despite awareness of interpersonal or social problems: *Do you use hallucinogens even though you suspect, or even know, that your use creates or worsens interpersonal or social problems?*

vii. Giving up activities for hallucinogens: *Are there important social, occupational, or recreational activities that you have given up or reduced because of your hallucinogen use?*

viii. Use in hazardous situations: *Have you repeatedly used hallucinogens in situations in which it was phys-*

ically hazardous, such as driving a car or operating a machine while intoxicated?

ix. Continued use despite awareness of physical or psychological problems: *Do you use hallucinogens even though you suspect, or even know, that they create or worsen problems with your mind and body?*

x. Tolerance as manifested by <u>either</u> of the following.

- Markedly increased amounts: *Do you find that to achieve the desired effect of hallucinogens you need to consume much more than you used to?*
- Markedly diminished effects: *If you use the same amount of a hallucinogen as you used to, do you find that it has a lot less effect on you than it used to?*

b. Modifiers

i. Specifiers

- In early remission
- In sustained remission
- In a controlled environment

ii. Severity

- Mild: Use when two or three criteria are present.
- Moderate: Use when four or five criteria are present.
- Severe: Use when six or more criteria are present.

c. Alternatives

i. If a young person reports reexperiencing perceptual symptoms they first experienced while impaired by a hallucinogen after ceasing use, consider hallucinogen persisting perception disorder (full criteria are in DSM-5-TR, p. 598). The symptoms must cause clinically significant distress or impairment.

ii. If a young person experiences problems associated with the use of phencyclidine or other hallucinogens that are not classifiable as phencyclidine or other hallucinogen use disorder, intoxication, withdrawal, intoxication delirium, withdrawal delirium, phencyclidine- or other hallucinogen-induced neurocognitive disorder, phencyclidine- or other hallucinogen-induced psychotic disorder, phencyclidine- or other hallucinogen-induced bipolar disorder, phencyclidine- or other hallucinogen-induced depressive disorder, phencyclidine- or other hallucinogen-induced anxiety disorder, phencyclidine- or other hallucinogen-induced sexual dysfunction, or phencyclidine- or other hallucinogen-induced sleep disorder, consider unspecified phencyclidine-related disorder (see DSM-5-TR, p. 600) or unspecified hallucinogen-related disorder (see DSM-5-TR, p. 601).

10. Phencyclidine Intoxication or Other Hallucinogen Intoxication

   a. Inclusion: Requires at least <u>two</u> of the following signs during or shortly after hallucinogen use.

   Phencyclidine

       i. Vertical or horizontal nystagmus
       ii. Hypertension or tachycardia
       iii. Numbness or diminished responsiveness to pain
       iv. Ataxia
       v. Dysarthria
       vi. Muscle rigidity
       vii. Seizures or coma
       viii. Hyperacusis

   Other Hallucinogens

       i. Pupillary dilation
       ii. Tachycardia
       iii. Sweating: *Since taking the hallucinogen, have you noticed any change in how much you sweat?*
       iv. Palpitations: *Since taking the hallucinogen, has your heartbeat been more rapid, strong, or irregular than usual?*
       v. Blurring of vision: *Since taking the hallucinogen, has your vision been blurred?*
       vi. Tremors
       vii. Incoordination: *Since taking the hallucinogen, have you found it hard to coordinate your movements as you walk or otherwise move?*

   b. Inclusion: Requires clinically significant problematic behavioral or psychological changes. *Since you began this episode of hallucinogen use, have you observed any significant changes in your mood, judgment, ability to inter-*

act with others, or sense of time? Have you engaged in problematic activities, or thought problematic thoughts, that you would not have without hallucinogens?

c. Exclusion: If the symptoms are attributable to another medical condition or are better explained by another mental disorder, including intoxication with another substance, do not make the diagnosis.

11. Inhalant Use Disorder

a. Inclusion: Requires a problematic pattern of inhalant use leading to clinically significant impairment or distress as manifested by at least <u>two</u> of the following in a 12-month period.

i. Using more inhalants over a longer period than intended: *When you inhale, do you find that you use more inhalant, and for a longer time, than you planned to?*

ii. Persistent desire or unsuccessful effort to reduce inhalant use: *Do you want to cut back or stop inhaling? Have you ever tried and failed to cut back or stop inhaling?*

iii. Great deal of time spent: *Do you spend a great deal of your time obtaining inhalants, using inhalants, or recovering from your inhalant use?*

iv. Cravings: *Do you experience strong desires or cravings to use inhalants?*

v. Failure to fulfill major role obligations: *Have you repeatedly failed to fulfill major obligations at home, school, or work because of your inhalant use?*

vi. Continued use despite awareness of interpersonal or social problems: *Do you use inhalants even though you suspect, or even know, that your use creates or worsens interpersonal or social problems?*

vii. Giving up activities for inhalants: *Are there important social, occupational, or recreational activities that you have given up or reduced because of your inhalant use?*

viii. Use in hazardous situations: *Have you repeatedly used inhalants in situations in which it was physically hazardous, such as driving a car or operating a machine while high?*

ix. Continued use despite awareness of physical or psychological problems: *Do you use inhalants even though you suspect, or even know, that it creates or worsens problems with your mind and body?*

x. Tolerance as manifested by <u>either</u> of the following.

- Markedly increased amounts: *Do you find that to get high or achieve the desired effect of using inhalants you need to use much more than you used to?*
- Markedly diminished effects: *If you inhale the same amount of an inhalant as you used to, do you find that it has a lot less effect on you than it used to?*

b. Modifiers

    i. Specifiers
- In early remission
- In sustained remission
- In a controlled environment

    ii. Severity
- Mild: Use when two or three criteria are present.
- Moderate: Use when four or five criteria are present.
- Severe: Use when six or more criteria are present.

c. Alternative: If a young person experiences problems associated with the use of an inhalant that are not classifiable as inhalant use disorder, intoxication, withdrawal, inhalant intoxication delirium, inhalant withdrawal delirium, inhalant-induced neurocognitive disorder, inhalant-induced psychotic disorder, inhalant-induced bipolar disorder, inhalant-induced depressive disorder, inhalant-induced anxiety disorder, inhalant-induced sexual dysfunction, or inhalant-induced sleep disorder, consider unspecified inhalant-related disorder (see DSM-5-TR, p. 608).

12. Inhalant Intoxication

a. Inclusion: Requires at least <u>two</u> of the following signs or symptoms after intended or unintended short-term, high-dose inhalant exposure.

    i. Dizziness: *Since using the inhalant, have you felt like you were reeling or about to fall?*

    ii. Nystagmus

    iii. Incoordination: *Since using the inhalant, have you found it hard to coordinate your movements as you walk or otherwise move?*

    iv. Slurred speech

    v. Unsteady gait

    vi.   Lethargy: *Since using the inhalant, have you felt very sleepy or felt a marked lack of energy?*

   vii.   Depressed reflexes

  viii.   Psychomotor retardation

    ix.   Tremor

     x.   Generalized muscle weakness

    xi.   Blurred vision or diplopia: *Since using the inhalant, has your vision been blurred, or have you been seeing double?*

   xii.   Stupor or coma

  xiii.   Euphoria: *Since using the inhalant, have you felt mentally or physically elated or intensely excited or happy?*

b.   Inclusion: Requires clinically significant problematic behavioral or psychological changes. *Since you began this episode of inhalant use, have you observed any significant changes in your mood, judgment, ability to interact with others, or sense of time? Have you engaged in problematic activities, or thought problematic thoughts, that you would not have without inhalants?*

c.   Exclusion: If the symptoms are attributable to another medical condition or are better explained by another mental disorder, including intoxication with another substance, do not make the diagnosis.

13. Opioid Use Disorder

a.   Inclusion: Requires a maladaptive pattern of opioid use leading to clinically significant impairment or distress as manifested by at least <u>two</u> of the following in a 12-month period.

     i.   Using more opioids over a longer period than intended: *When you use opioids, do you find that you use more, and for a longer time, than you planned to?*

    ii.   Persistent desire or unsuccessful effort to reduce opioid use: *Do you want to cut back or stop using opioids? Have you ever tried and failed to cut back or stop your opioid use?*

   iii.   Great deal of time spent: *Do you spend a great deal of your time obtaining opioids, using opioids, or recovering from your opioid use?*

    iv.   Cravings: *Do you experience strong desires or cravings to use opioids?*

     v.   Failure to fulfill major role obligations: *Have you repeatedly failed to fulfill major obligations at home, school, or work because of your opioid use?*

vi.   Continued use despite awareness of interpersonal or social problems: *Do you continue to use opioids even though you suspect, or even know, that your use creates or worsens interpersonal or social problems?*

vii. Giving up activities for opioids: *Are there important social, occupational, or recreational activities that you have given up or reduced because of your opioid use?*

viii. Use in hazardous situations: *Have you repeatedly used opioids in situations in which it was physically hazardous, such as driving a car or operating a machine while intoxicated?*

ix.   Continued use despite awareness of physical or psychological problems: *Do you use opioids even though you suspect, or even know, that it creates or worsens problems with your mind and body?*

x.   Tolerance as manifested by <u>either</u> of the following.

- Markedly increased amounts: *Do you find that to get high or achieve the desired effect of using opioids you need to consume much more than you used to?*

- Markedly diminished effects (excluding opioid medications taken under medical supervision): *If you use the same amount of an opioid as you used to, do you find that it has a lot less effect on you than it used to?*

xi.   Withdrawal as manifested by <u>either</u> of the following.

- Characteristic opioid withdrawal syndrome: *When you stop using opioids, do you undergo withdrawal?*

- The same or a closely related substance is taken to relieve or avoid withdrawal symptoms: *Have you ever taken opioids or another substance to prevent opioid withdrawal?*

b. Modifiers

i. Specifiers

- In early remission
- In sustained remission
- On maintenance therapy
- In a controlled environment

    ii. Severity

- Mild: Use when two or three criteria are present.
- Moderate: Use when four or five criteria are present.
- Severe: Use when six or more criteria are present.

c. Alternative: If a young person experiences problems associated with the use of opioids that are not classifiable as opioid use disorder, intoxication, withdrawal, intoxication delirium, withdrawal delirium, opioid-induced neurocognitive disorder, opioid-induced psychotic disorder, opioid-induced bipolar disorder, opioid-induced depressive disorder, opioid-induced anxiety disorder, opioid-induced sexual dysfunction, or opioid-induced sleep disorder, consider unspecified opioid-related disorder (see DSM-5-TR, p. 619).

14. Opioid Intoxication

a. Inclusion: Requires pupillary constriction shortly after opioid use and at least <u>one</u> of the following signs.

    i. Drowsiness or coma
    ii. Slurred speech
    iii. Impairment in attention or memory

b. Inclusion: Requires clinically significant problematic behavioral or psychological changes. *Since you began this episode of opioid use, have you observed any significant changes in your mood, judgment, ability to interact with others, or sense of time? Have you engaged in problematic activities, or thought problematic thoughts, that you would not have without opioids?*

c. Exclusion: If the symptoms are attributable to another medical condition or are better explained by another mental disorder, including intoxication with another substance, do not make the diagnosis.

d. Modifiers

    i. Specifier

- With perceptual disturbance: Use when hallucinations occur with intact reality testing or when auditory, visual, or tactile illusions occur in the absence of delirium.

15. Opioid Withdrawal

   a. Inclusion: Requires at least <u>three</u> of the following symptoms developing within minutes to several days of ceasing (or reducing) opioid use that has been heavy and prolonged *or* following the administration of an opioid antagonist after a period of opioid use.

      i. Dysphoric mood: *Over the past couple of days, have you been feeling more down or depressed than usual?*

      ii. Nausea or vomiting: *Over the past couple of days, have you felt sick to your stomach, felt nauseated, or even vomited?*

      iii. Muscle aches: *Over the past couple of days, have you experienced muscle aches or pains?*

      iv. Lacrimation or rhinorrhea: *Over the past couple of days, have you noticed that you have been shedding tears when you did not feel like crying? Have you noticed that your nose has been running, or discharging clear fluid, more than usual?*

      v. Pupillary dilation, piloerection, or sweating

      vi. Diarrhea: *Over the past couple of days, have you experienced more frequent or more liquid stools than usual?*

      vii. Yawning: *Over the past couple of days, have you been yawning much more than usual?*

      viii. Fever

      ix. Insomnia: *Over the past couple of days, have you found it more difficult than usual to get to sleep and to stay asleep?*

   b. Exclusion: If the symptoms are attributable to another medical condition or are better explained by another mental disorder, including intoxication with or withdrawal from another substance, do not make the diagnosis.

16. Sedative, Hypnotic, or Anxiolytic Use Disorder

   a. Inclusion: Requires a problematic pattern of sedative, hypnotic, or anxiolytic use leading to clinically significant impairment or distress as manifested by at least <u>two</u> of the following in a 12-month period.

      i. Using more sedatives, hypnotics, or anxiolytics over a longer period than intended: *When you use sedatives, hypnotics, or anxiolytics, do you find that you use more, and for a longer time, than you planned to?*

ii. Persistent desire or unsuccessful effort to reduce sedative, hypnotic, or anxiolytic use: *Do you want to cut back or stop using sedatives, hypnotics, or anxiolytics? Have you ever tried and failed to cut back or stop using sedatives, hypnotics, or anxiolytics?*

iii. Great deal of time spent: *Do you spend a great deal of your time obtaining and using sedatives, hypnotics, or anxiolytics or recovering from your sedative, hypnotic, or anxiolytic use?*

iv. Cravings: *Do you experience strong desires or cravings to use sedatives, hypnotics, or anxiolytics?*

v. Failure to fulfill major role obligations: *Have you repeatedly failed to fulfill major obligations at home, school, or work because of your sedative, hypnotic, or anxiolytic use?*

vi. Continued use despite awareness of interpersonal or social problems: *Do you use a sedative, hypnotic, or anxiolytic even though you suspect, or even know, that it creates or worsens interpersonal or social problems?*

vii. Giving up activities for sedatives, hypnotics, or anxiolytics: *Are there important social, occupational, or recreational activities that you have given up or reduced because of your sedative, hypnotic, or anxiolytic use?*

viii. Use in hazardous situations: *Have you repeatedly used a sedative, hypnotic, or anxiolytic in situations in which it was physically hazardous, such as driving a car or operating a machine while intoxicated?*

ix. Continued use despite awareness of physical or psychological problems: *Do you use sedatives, hypnotics, or anxiolytics even though you suspect, or even know, that your use creates or worsens problems with your mind and body?*

x. Tolerance as manifested by <u>either</u> of the following.
   - Markedly increased amounts: *Do you find that to get intoxicated or achieve the desired effect of using sedatives, hypnotics, or anxiolytics you need to consume much more than you used to?*
   - Markedly diminished effects: *If you use the same amount of a sedative, hypnotic, or anxiolytic as you used to, do you find that it has a lot less effect on you than it used to?*

xi. Withdrawal as manifested by <u>either</u> of the following.
   - Characteristic sedative, hypnotic, or anxiolytic withdrawal syndrome: *When you stop using*

sedatives, hypnotics, or anxiolytics, do you undergo withdrawal?
- The same or a closely related substance is taken to relieve or avoid withdrawal symptoms: *Have you ever taken sedatives, hypnotics, anxiolytics, or another substance to prevent withdrawal?*

b. Modifiers

   i. Specifiers

   - In early remission
   - In sustained remission
   - In a controlled environment

   ii. Severity

   - Mild: Use when two or three criteria are present.
   - Moderate: Use when four or five criteria are present.
   - Severe: Use when six or more criteria are present.

c. Alternative: If a young person experiences problems associated with the use of a sedative, hypnotic, or anxiolytic that are not classifiable as sedative, hypnotic, or anxiolytic use disorder, intoxication, withdrawal, or delirium; or experiences problems associated with but not classifiable as sedative-, hypnotic-, or anxiolytic-induced neurocognitive disorder, psychotic disorder, anxiety disorder, or sleep disorder, then consider unspecified sedative-, hypnotic-, or anxiolytic-related disorder (see DSM-5-TR, p. 632).

17. Sedative, Hypnotic, or Anxiolytic Intoxication

a. Inclusion: Requires <u>one</u> of the following signs shortly after sedative, hypnotic, or anxiolytic use.

   i. Slurred speech
   ii. Incoordination
   iii. Unsteady gait
   iv. Nystagmus
   v. Impairment in cognition (i.e., attention or memory)
   vi. Stupor or coma

b. Inclusion: Requires clinically significant problematic behavioral or psychological changes. *Since you began this episode of sedative, hypnotic, or anxiolytic use, have* you observed any significant changes in your mood, judgment, ability to interact with others, or sense of time? Have you engaged in problematic activities, or thought problematic thoughts, that you would not have without the sedative, hypnotic, or anxiolytic?

c. Exclusion: If the symptoms are attributable to another medical condition or are better explained by another mental disorder, including intoxication with another substance, do not make the diagnosis.

18. Sedative, Hypnotic, or Anxiolytic Withdrawal

a. Inclusion: Requires at least <u>two</u> of the following symptoms developing within several hours to a few days after ceasing (or reducing) sedative, hypnotic, or anxiolytic use that has been heavy and prolonged.

   i. Autonomic hyperactivity
   ii. Hand tremor
   iii. Insomnia: *Over the past couple of days, have you found it more difficult than usual to get to sleep and to stay asleep?*
   iv. Nausea or vomiting: *Over the past couple of days, have you felt sick to your stomach, felt nauseated, or even vomited?*
   v. Transient visual, tactile, or auditory hallucinations or illusions: *Over the past couple of days, have you had any experiences where you worried that your mind was playing tricks on you, like seeing, hearing, or feeling things that other people could not?*
   vi. Psychomotor agitation
   vii. Anxiety: *Over the past couple of days, have you felt more worried or anxious than usual?*
   viii. Grand mal seizures

b. Exclusion: If the symptoms are attributable to another medical condition or are better explained by another mental disorder, including intoxication with or withdrawal from another substance, do not make the diagnosis.

c. Modifiers

   i. Specifier
      • With perceptual disturbance: Use when hallucinations occur with intact reality testing or when auditory, visual, or tactile illusions occur in the absence of delirium.

19. Stimulant Use Disorder

    a. Inclusion: Requires a problematic pattern of stimulant use leading to clinically significant impairment or distress as manifested by at least <u>two</u> of the following in a 12-month period.

        i. Using more stimulants over a longer period than intended: *When you use stimulants, do you find that you use more, and for a longer time, than you planned to?*

        ii. Persistent desire or unsuccessful effort to reduce stimulant use: *Do you want to cut back or stop using stimulants? Have you ever tried and failed to cut back or stop using stimulants?*

        iii. Great deal of time spent: *Do you spend a great deal of your time obtaining stimulants, using stimulants, or recovering from your stimulant use?*

        iv. Cravings: *Do you experience strong desires or cravings to use stimulants?*

        v. Failure to fulfill major role obligations: *Have you repeatedly failed to fulfill major obligations at home, school, or work because of your stimulant use?*

        vi. Continued use despite awareness of interpersonal or social problems: *Do you use stimulants even though you suspect, or even know, that your use creates or worsens interpersonal or social problems?*

        vii. Giving up activities for stimulants: *Are there important social, occupational, or recreational activities that you have given up or reduced because of your stimulant use?*

        viii. Use in hazardous situations: *Have you repeatedly used stimulants in situations in which it was physically hazardous, such as driving a car or operating a machine while intoxicated?*

        ix. Continued use despite awareness of physical or psychological problems: *Do you use stimulants even though you suspect, or even know, that it creates or worsens problems with your mind and body?*

        x. Tolerance as manifested by <u>either</u> of the following. **Note:** This criterion is not met if the young person is taking stimulants as prescribed under medical supervision.

            • Markedly increased amounts: *Do you find that to get intoxicated or achieve the desired effect of using stimulants you need to consume much more than you used to?*

- Markedly diminished effects (excluding stimulant medications taken under medical supervision to treat ADHD or narcolepsy): *If you use the same amount of a stimulant as you used to, do you find that it has a lot less effect on you than it used to?*

xi. Withdrawal as manifested by <u>either</u> of the following. **Note:** This criterion is not met if the young person is taking stimulants as prescribed under medical supervision.

- Characteristic stimulant withdrawal syndrome: *When you stop using stimulants, do you undergo withdrawal?*
- The same or a closely related substance is taken to relieve or avoid withdrawal symptoms (excluding stimulant medications taken under medical supervision to treat ADHD or narcolepsy): *Have you ever taken stimulants or another substance to prevent withdrawal?*

b. Modifiers

i. Specify stimulant

- Amphetamine-type substance
- Cocaine
- Other or unspecified stimulant

ii. Specifiers

- In early remission
- In sustained remission
- In a controlled environment

iii. Severity

- Mild: Use when two or three criteria are present.
- Moderate: Use when four or five criteria are present.
- Severe: Use when six or more criteria are present.

c. Alternative: If a young person experiences problems associated with the use of stimulants that are not classifiable as stimulant use disorder, intoxication, withdrawal, intoxication delirium, withdrawal delirium, stimulant-induced neurocognitive disorder, stimulant-induced psychotic disorder, stimulant-induced bipolar disorder, stimulant-induced depressive disorder, stimulant-induced anxiety disorder, stimulant-induced sexual dysfunction, or stimulant-induced sleep disorder, consider unspecified stimulant-related disorder (see DSM-5-TR, p. 644).

20. Stimulant Intoxication

   a. Inclusion: Requires at least <u>two</u> of the following signs shortly after stimulant use.

      i. Tachycardia or bradycardia
      ii. Pupillary dilation
      iii. Elevated or lowered blood pressure
      iv. Perspiration or chills: *Over the past couple of hours, have you experienced chills or been sweating more than usual?*
      v. Nausea or vomiting: *Over the past couple of hours, have you felt sick to your stomach, felt nauseated, or even vomited?*
      vi. Evidence of weight loss
      vii. Psychomotor agitation or retardation
      viii. Muscular weakness, respiratory depression, chest pain, or cardiac arrhythmias
      ix. Confusion, seizures, dyskinesias, dystonias, or coma

   b. Inclusion: Requires clinically significant problematic behavioral or psychological changes. *Since you began this episode of stimulant use, have you observed any significant changes in your mood, judgment, ability to interact with others, or sense of time? Have you engaged in problematic activities, or thought problematic thoughts, that you would not have without stimulants?*

   c. Exclusion: If the symptoms are attributable to another medical condition or are better explained by another mental disorder, including intoxication with another substance, do not make the diagnosis.

   d. Modifiers

      i. Specifiers

         • Specify the intoxicant: amphetamine, cocaine, or other stimulant
         • With perceptual disturbance: Use when hallucinations occur with intact reality testing or when auditory, visual, or tactile illusions occur in the absence of delirium.

21. Stimulant Withdrawal

  a. Inclusion: Requires the following symptom developing within hours to days of ceasing (or reducing) stimulant use that has been heavy or prolonged.

    i. Dysphoric mood: *Over the past few hours or days, have you felt much more down or depressed than usual?*

  b. Inclusion: Also requires at least <u>two</u> of the following symptoms developing simultaneously.

    i. Fatigue: *Over the past few hours or days, have you felt extremely sleepy or tired?*

    ii. Vivid, unpleasant dreams: *Over the past few hours or days, have you experienced unusually vivid, unpleasant dreams?*

    iii. Insomnia or hypersomnia: *Over the past few hours or days, have you found it more difficult than usual to get to sleep and to stay asleep? Alternatively, have you found that you have been sleeping much more than usual?*

    iv. Increased appetite: *Over the past few hours or days, have you desired food much more than usual?*

    v. Psychomotor retardation or agitation

  c. Exclusion: If the symptoms are attributable to another medical condition or are better explained by another mental disorder, including intoxication with or withdrawal from another substance, do not make the diagnosis.

  d. Modifiers

    i. Specifiers

      • Amphetamine-type substance, cocaine, or other stimulant

  e. Alternative: If a young person experiences problems associated with the use of a stimulant that are not classifiable as a stimulant-related disorder, consider unspecified stimulant-related disorder (see DSM-5-TR, p. 644).

22. Tobacco Use Disorder

  a. Inclusion: Requires a problematic pattern of tobacco use leading to clinically significant impairment or distress as manifested by at least <u>two</u> of the following in a 12-month period.

i. Using more tobacco over a longer period than intended: *When you use tobacco, do you find that you use more, and for a longer time, than you planned to?*

ii. Persistent desire or unsuccessful effort to reduce tobacco use: *Do you want to cut back or stop using tobacco? Have you ever tried and failed to cut back or stop using tobacco?*

iii. Great deal of time spent: *Do you spend a great deal of your time obtaining tobacco, using tobacco, or recovering from your tobacco use?*

iv. Cravings: *Do you experience strong desires or cravings to use tobacco?*

v. Failure to fulfill major role obligations: *Have you repeatedly failed to fulfill major obligations at home, school, or work because of your tobacco use?*

vi. Continued use despite awareness of interpersonal or social problems: *Do you use tobacco even though you suspect, or even know, that your use creates or worsens interpersonal or social problems?*

vii. Giving up activities for tobacco: *Are there important social, occupational, or recreational activities that you have given up or reduced because of your tobacco use?*

viii. Use in hazardous situations: *Have you repeatedly used tobacco in situations in which it was physically hazardous, such as smoking in bed?*

ix. Continued use despite awareness of physical or psychological problems: *Do you use tobacco even though you suspect, or even know, that it creates or worsens problems with your mind and body?*

x. Tolerance as manifested by either of the following.

- Markedly increased amounts: *Do you find that to get the desired effect of tobacco you need to consume much more than you used to?*

- Markedly diminished effects: *If you use the same amount of tobacco as you used to, do you find that it has a lot less effect on you than it used to?*

xi. Withdrawal as manifested by either of the following.

- Characteristic tobacco withdrawal syndrome: *When you stop using tobacco, do you undergo withdrawal?*

- The same substance is taken to relieve or avoid withdrawal symptoms: *Have you ever used to-*

bacco to avoid or relieve symptoms of tobacco withdrawal?

b. Modifiers

i. Specifiers

- In early remission
- In sustained remission
- On maintenance therapy
- In a controlled environment

ii. Severity

- Mild: Use when two or three criteria are present.
- Moderate: Use when four or five criteria are present.
- Severe: Use when six or more criteria are present.

c. Alternative: If a young person experiences clinically significant problems associated with the use of to-bacco that do not meet criteria for a specific diagnosis, consider unspecified tobacco-related disorder (see DSM-5-TR, p. 651).

23. Tobacco Withdrawal

a. Inclusion: Requires at least <u>four</u> of the following symptoms developing within 24 hours of ceasing (or reducing) tobacco use that has been daily for at least several weeks.

i. Irritability, frustration, or anger: *Over the past 24 hours, have you felt more irritable, frustrated, or angry than usual?*

ii. Anxiety: *Over the past 24 hours, have you felt more worried or anxious than usual?*

iii. Difficulty concentrating: *Over the past 24 hours, have you had difficulty staying focused on a task or an activity?*

iv. Increased appetite: *Over the past 24 hours, have you desired food more than usual?*

v. Restlessness: *Over the past 24 hours, have you felt less able to remain at rest than usual?*

vi. Depressed mood: *Over the past 24 hours, have you been feeling more down or depressed than usual?*

vii. Insomnia: *Over the past 24 hours, have you found it more difficult than usual to get to sleep and to stay asleep?*

b. Exclusion: If the symptoms are attributable to another medical condition or are better explained by another mental disorder, including intoxication with or withdrawal from another substance, do not make the diagnosis.

c. Alternative: If a person experiences problems associated with the use of a tobacco-related disorder that does not meet the criteria for tobacco withdrawal, consider unspecified tobacco related disorder (see DSM-5-TR, p. 651).

24. Other (or Unknown) Substance Use Disorder

a. Inclusion: Requires a problematic pattern of use of an intoxicating substance not able to be classified within the other substance categories listed earlier in this section, leading to clinically significant impairment or distress as manifested by at least <u>two</u> of the following in a 12-month period.

    i. Taking more of the substance over a longer period than intended: *When you use the substance, do you find that you use it more often, or for a longer time, than you planned to?*

    ii. Persistent desire or unsuccessful effort to reduce substance use: *Do you want to cut back or stop using the substance? Have you ever tried and failed to cut back or stop using the substance?*

    iii. Great deal of time spent: *Do you spend a great deal of your time obtaining or using the substance or recovering from your substance use?*

    iv. Cravings: *Do you experience strong desires or cravings to use the substance?*

    v. Failure to fulfill major role obligations: *Have you repeatedly failed to fulfill major obligations at home, school, or work because of your substance use?*

    vi. Continued use despite awareness of interpersonal or social problems: *Do you use the substance even though you suspect, or even know, that it creates or worsens interpersonal or social problems?*

    vii. Giving up activities for the substance: *Are there important social, occupational, or recreational activities that you have given up or reduced because of your substance use?*

    viii. Use in hazardous situations: *Have you repeatedly used the substance in situations in which it was physi-*

cally hazardous, such as driving a car or operating a machine while intoxicated?

ix. Continued use despite awareness of physical or psychological problems: *Do you use the substance even though you suspect, or even know, that it creates or worsens problems with your mind and body?*

x. Tolerance as manifested by <u>either</u> of the following.

- Markedly increased amounts: *Do you find that to get intoxicated or achieve the desired effect of substance use you need to consume much more of the substance than you used to?*
- Markedly diminished effects: *If you use the same amount of the substance as you used to, do you find that it has a lot less effect on you than it used to?*

xi. Withdrawal as manifested by <u>either</u> of the following.

- Characteristic withdrawal syndrome for the substance: *When you stop using the substance, do you undergo withdrawal?*
- The same or a closely related substance is taken to relieve or avoid withdrawal symptoms: *Have you ever taken the substance or another substance to prevent withdrawal?*

b. Modifiers

i. Specifiers

- In early remission
- In sustained remission
- In a controlled environment

ii. Severity

- Mild: Use when two or three criteria are present.
- Moderate: Use when four or five criteria are present.
- Severe: Use when six or more criteria are present.

25. Other (or Unknown) Substance Intoxication

a. Inclusion: Development of a reversible substance-specific syndrome attributable to recent ingestion of (or exposure to) a substance that is not listed elsewhere in this section or is unknown.

b. Inclusion: Requires clinically significant problematic behavioral or psychological changes. *Since you began using this substance, have you observed any significant changes in your mood, judgment, ability to interact with others, or sense of time? Have you engaged in problematic activities, or thought problematic thoughts, that you would not have without using this substance?*

c. Exclusion: If the symptoms are attributable to another medical condition or are better explained by another mental disorder, including intoxication with another substance, do not make the diagnosis.

26. Other (or Unknown) Substance Withdrawal

   a. Inclusion: Development of a substance-specific syndrome shortly after the cessation of (or a reduction in) use of the substance that has been heavy and prolonged.

   b. Inclusion: Requires clinically significant distress or impairment in social, occupational, or other important areas of functioning.

   c. Exclusion: If the symptoms are attributable to another medical condition or are better explained by another mental disorder, including withdrawal from another substance, do not make the diagnosis.

27. Gambling Disorder

   a. Inclusion: Requires persistent, recurrent problematic gambling that leads to clinically significant impairment or distress, lasting at least 12 months, as indicated by at least <u>four</u> of the following symptoms.

      i. Escalates spending on gambling: *Do you find that it takes increasing amounts of money to get the excitement you want from gambling?*

      ii. Is irritable when quitting: *When you try to reduce or quit gambling, are you irritable or restless?*

      iii. Is unable to quit: *Have you unsuccessfully tried to reduce or quit gambling on several occasions?*

      iv. Is preoccupied: *Are you preoccupied with gambling?*

      v. Gambles when distressed: *When you are feeling anxious, down, or helpless, do you gamble?*

      vi. Chases losses: *After you lose money, do you return another day to try to get even?*

      vii. Lies: *Do you lie to conceal how much you gamble?*

      viii. Loses relationships: *Have you lost a relationship, job, or opportunity because of your gambling?*

      ix. Borrows money: *Do you rely on other people for*

> *money to cover desperate financial situations caused by gambling?*

b. Exclusion: If the gambling behavior is better accounted for by a manic episode, do not make the diagnosis.

c. Modifiers

   i. Course

   - Episodic: Experiencing symptoms that meet diagnostic criteria at more than one time point, with symptoms subsiding between periods of gambling disorder for at least several months
   - Persistent: Experiencing continuous symptoms that meet diagnostic criteria for multiple years
   - In early remission
   - In sustained remission

   ii. Severity

   - Mild: Use when four or five criteria are present.
   - Moderate: Use when six or seven criteria are present.
   - Severe: Use when eight or nine criteria are present.

Medication-Induced Movement Disorders and Other Adverse Effects of Medication

DSM-5-TR pp. 807–819

Medication-Induced Movement Disorders

- G21.11   Antipsychotic medication and other dopamine receptor blocking agent–induced parkinsonism
- G21.19   Other medication-induced parkinsonism
- G21.0   Neuroleptic malignant syndrome
- G24.02   Medication-induced acute dystonia
- G25.71   Medication-induced acute akathisia
- G24.01   Tardive dyskinesia
- G24.09   Tardive dystonia
- G25.71   Tardive akathisia

- G25.1   Medication-induced postural tremor
- G25.79   Other medication-induced movement disorder

Antidepressant Discontinuation Syndrome

- T43.205A   Initial encounter
- T43.205D   Subsequent encounter
- T43.205S   Sequelae

Other Adverse Effect of Medication

- T50.905A   Initial encounter
- T50.905D   Subsequent encounter
- T50.905S   Sequelae

Other Conditions That May Be a Focus of Clinical Attention

DSM-5-TR pp. 821–836

A patient's mental disorder is affected by the other conditions and any psychosocial or environmental problems they have. To assist a clinician addressing the other conditions that alter the diagnosis, course, prognosis, and treatment of a patient's mental disorder, DSM-5-TR provides a list of selected conditions and problems drawn from ICD-10-CM (usually Z codes). A condition or problem listed here may be coded if it is initiated or exacerbated by a mental disorder; is a reason for the current visit; constitutes a problem that must be considered for the overall management; or otherwise helps explain the need for a test, procedure, or treatment.

Conditions and problems from this list may also be included in the medical record as useful information on circumstances that may affect the patient's care, regardless of their relevance to the current visit. The conditions and problems listed here are not mental disorders. Their inclusion in DSM-5-TR is meant to draw attention to the scope of additional issues that are encountered in routine clinical practice and to provide a systematic listing that may be useful to clinicians in documenting these issues.

Suicidal Behavior and Nonsuicidal Self-Injury

Suicidal Behavior

Current Suicidal Behavior

- T14.91XA   Initial encounter
- T14.91XD   Subsequent encounter
- Z91.51   History of Suicidal Behavior

Nonsuicidal Self-Injury

- R45.88   Current Nonsuicidal Self-Injury
- Z91.52   History of Nonsuicidal Self-Injury

Abuse and Neglect

Child Maltreatment and Neglect Problems

Child Physical Abuse

Child Physical Abuse, Confirmed

- T74.12XA   Initial encounter
- T74.12XD   Subsequent encounter

Child Physical Abuse, Suspected

- T76.12XA   Initial encounter
- T76.12XD   Subsequent encounter

Other Circumstances Related to Child Physical Abuse

- Z69.010   Encounter for mental health services for victim of child physical abuse by parent
- Z69.020   Encounter for mental health services for victim of nonparental child physical abuse
- Z62.810   Personal history (past history) of physical abuse in childhood
- Z69.011   Encounter for mental health services for perpetrator of parental child physical abuse
- Z69.021   Encounter for mental health services for perpetrator of nonparental child physical abuse

Child Sexual Abuse

Child Sexual Abuse, Confirmed

- T74.22XA   Initial encounter
- T74.22XD   Subsequent encounter

Child Sexual Abuse, Suspected

- T76.22XA   Initial encounter
- T76.22XD   Subsequent encounter

Other Circumstances Related to Child Sexual Abuse

- Z69.010   Encounter for mental health services for victim of child sexual abuse by parent
- Z69.020   Encounter for mental health services for victim of nonparental child sexual abuse
- Z62.810   Personal history (past history) of sexual abuse in childhood
- Z69.011   Encounter for mental health services for perpetrator of parental child sexual abuse
- Z69.021   Encounter for mental health services for perpetrator of nonparental child sexual abuse

Child Neglect

Child Neglect, Confirmed

- T74.02XA   Initial encounter
- T74.02XD   Subsequent encounter

Child Neglect, Suspected

- T76.02XA   Initial encounter
- T76.02XD   Subsequent encounter

Other Circumstances Related to Child Neglect

- Z69.010   Encounter for mental health services for victim of child neglect by parent
- Z69.020   Encounter for mental health services for victim of nonparental child neglect

- Z62.812   Personal history (past history) of neglect in childhood
- Z69.011   Encounter for mental health services for perpetrator of parental child neglect
- Z69.021   Encounter for mental health services for perpetrator of nonparental child neglect

Child Psychological Abuse

Child Psychological Abuse, Confirmed

- T74.32XA   Initial encounter
- T74.32XD   Subsequent encounter

Child Psychological Abuse, Suspected

- T76.32XA   Initial encounter
- T76.32XD   Subsequent encounter

Other Circumstances Related to Child Psychological Abuse

- Z69.010   Encounter for mental health services for victim of child psychological abuse by parent
- Z69.020   Encounter for mental health services for victim of nonparental child psychological abuse
- Z62.811   Personal history (past history) of psychological abuse in childhood
- Z69.011   Encounter for mental health services for perpetrator of parental child psychological abuse
- Z69.021   Encounter for mental health services for perpetrator of nonparental child psychological abuse

Relational Problems

Parent-Child Relational Problem

- Z62.820   Parent–Biological Child
- Z62.821   Parent–Adopted Child
- Z62.822   Parent–Foster Child
- Z62.898   Other Caregiver–Child
- Z62.891   Sibling Relational Problem
- Z63.0   Relationship Distress With Spouse or Intimate Partner

Problems Related to the Family Environment

- Z62.29   Upbringing Away From Parents
- Z62.898   Child Affected by Parental Relationship Distress
- Z63.5   Disruption of Family by Separation or Divorce
- Z63.8   High Expressed Emotion Level Within Family

Educational Problems

- Z55.0   Illiteracy and Low-Level Literacy
- Z55.1   Schooling Unavailable and Unattainable
- Z55.2   Failed School Examinations
- Z55.3   Underachievement in School
- Z55.4   Educational Maladjustment and Discord With Teachers and Classmates
- Z55.8   Problems Related to Inadequate Teaching
- Z55.9   Other Problems Related to Education and Literacy

Occupational Problems

- Z56.82   Problem Related to Current Military Deployment Status
- Z56.0   Unemployment
- Z56.1   Change of Job
- Z56.2   Threat of Job Loss
- Z56.3   Stressful Work Schedule
- Z56.4   Discord With Boss and Workmates
- Z56.5   Uncongenial Work Environment
- Z56.6   Other Physical and Mental Strain Related to Work
- Z56.81   Sexual Harassment on the Job
- Z56.9   Other Problem Related to Employment

Housing Problems

- Z59.01   Sheltered Homelessness
- Z59.02   Unsheltered Homelessness
- Z59.1   Inadequate Housing
- Z59.2   Discord With Neighbor, Lodger, or Landlord
- Z59.3   Problem Related to Living in a Residential Institution
- Z59.9   Other Housing Problem

Economic Problems

- Z59.41 Food Insecurity
- Z58.6 Lack of Safe Drinking Water
- Z59.5 Extreme Poverty
- Z59.6 Low Income
- Z59.7 Insufficient Social or Health Insurance or Welfare Support
- Z59.9 Other Economic Problem

Problems Related to the Social Environment

- Z60.2 Problem Related to Living Alone
- Z60.3 Acculturation Difficulty
- Z60.4 Social Exclusion or Rejection
- Z60.5 Target of (Perceived) Adverse Discrimination or Persecution
- Z60.9 Other Problem Related to Social Environment

Problems Related to Interaction With the Legal System

- Z65.0 Conviction in Civil or Criminal Proceedings Without Imprisonment
- Z65.1 Imprisonment or Other Incarceration
- Z65.2 Problems Related to Release From Prison
- Z65.3 Problems Related to Other Legal Circumstances

Problems Related to Other Psychosocial, Personal, and Environmental Circumstances

- Z72.9 Problem Related to Lifestyle
- Z64.0 Problems Related to Unwanted Pregnancy
- Z64.1 Problems Related to Multiparity
- Z64.4 Discord With Social Service Provider, Including Probation Officer, Case Manager, or Social Services Worker
- Z65.4 Victim of Crime
- Z65.4 Victim of Terrorism or Torture
- Z65.5 Exposure to Disaster, War, or Other Hostilities

Problems Related to Access to Medical and Other Health Care

- Z75.3 Unavailability or Inaccessibility of Health Care Facilities
- Z75.4 Unavailability or Inaccessibility of Other Helping Agencies

Circumstances of Personal History

- Z91.49 Personal History of Psychological Trauma
- Z91.82 Personal History of Military Deployment

Other Health Service Encounters for Counseling and Medical Advice

- Z31.5 Genetic Counseling
- Z70.9 Sex Counseling
- Z71.3 Dietary Counseling
- Z71.9 Other Counseling or Consultation

Additional Conditions or Problems That May Be a Focus of Clinical Attention

- Z91.83 Wandering Associated With a Mental Disorder
- Z63.4 Uncomplicated Bereavement
- Z60.0 Phase of Life Problem
- Z65.8 Religious or Spiritual Problem
- Z72.810 Child or Adolescent Antisocial Behavior
- Z91.199 Nonadherence to Medical Treatment
- E66.9 Overweight or Obesity
- Z76.5 Malingering
- R41.83 Borderline Intellectual Functioning

Symptoms and Signs Involving Emotional States

- R45.0 Nervousness
- R45.1 Relentlessness and agitation
- R45.2 Unhappiness
- R45.3 Demoralization and apathy

- R45.4   Irritability and anger
- R45.5   Hostility
- R45.6   Violent behavior
- R45.7   State of emotional shock and stress, unspecified
- R45.8   Other symptoms and signs involving emotional state
  - R45.81   Low self esteem
  - R45.82   Worries
  - R45.83   Excessive crying
  - R45.84   Anhedonia
  - R45.85   Homicidal and suicidal ideations
  - R45.850   Homicidal ideations
  - R45.851   Suicidal ideations
  - R45.86   Emotional lability
  - R45.87   Impulsiveness
  - R45.88   Nonsuicidal self-harm
  - R45.89   Other symptoms and signs involving emotional state

Chapter 8

Recalling Common DSM-5-TR Diagnoses Through Tables

TABLE 8–1. Abbreviated DSM-5-TR criteria for common diagnoses

Diagnosis	Criteria/time	Symptoms
Neurodevelopmental disorders		
ADHD	≥6 for ≥6 months *OR*	Inattention: makes careless mistakes; cannot sustain attention; does not seem to listen; often does not follow through; struggles to organize tasks; dislikes sustained mental effort; loses objects necessary for tasks; distracted by extraneous stimuli; forgetful in daily activities
	≥6 for ≥6 months	Hyperactivity/impulsivity: fidgets; leaves seat when sitting is expected; runs or climbs when inappropriate; unable to remain quiet; on the go as if driven by a motor; talks excessively; blurts out answers; cannot wait turn; interrupts; acts without thinking
Intellectual disability	Both beginning in early childhood	Deficits in intellectual functions confirmed by clinical assessment and standardized intelligence testing; deficits in adaptive functioning
Autism spectrum disorder	All 3 in multiple contexts, beginning in early childhood *AND*	Deficits in social-emotional reciprocity; deficits in nonverbal communicative behaviors; deficits in developing and maintaining relationships

TABLE 8-1. Abbreviated DSM-5-TR criteria for common diagnoses *(continued)*

Diagnosis	Criteria/time	Symptoms
	≥2	Stereotyped or repetitive motor movements, use of objects, or speech; inflexible adherence to routines or excessive resistance to change; highly restricted, fixated interests of abnormal intensity or focus; hyperreactivity or hyporeactivity to sensory input
Specific learning disorder	≥1 for ≥6 months beginning during childhood *DESPITE* interventions to reduce difficulties	Inaccurate or slow word reading; impaired reading comprehension; difficulties with spelling; difficulties with written expression; difficulties with number sense or calculations; difficulties with mathematical reasoning
Schizophrenia spectrum and other psychotic disorders		
Schizophrenia	≥2 for ≥1 month *AND*	Delusions; hallucinations; disorganized speech; grossly disorganized or catatonic behavior; negative symptoms (at least one symptom is delusions, hallucinations, or disorganized speech)
	≥6 months	Continuous signs of disturbance
Schizoaffective disorder	≥50% of the time *AND*	Criteria for schizophrenia

TABLE 8–1. Abbreviated DSM-5-TR criteria for common diagnoses (*continued*)

Diagnosis	Criteria/time	Symptoms
Schizophrenia spectrum and other psychotic disorders (*continued*)		
Schizoaffective disorder (*continued*)	≥2 weeks	Also experiences major depressive or manic episodes
		Delusions or hallucinations without depressive or manic episodes
Bipolar and related disorders		
Bipolar I disorder	≥1 week (or any duration if hospitalized) *AND*	Mania: abnormally, persistently elevated or irritable mood; persistently increased energy or activity, in a clear change from baseline energy or activity
	≥3	Inflated self-esteem or grandiosity; decreased need for sleep; pressured speech; flight of ideas or racing thoughts; distractibility; increase in goal-directed activity; excessive involvement in activities with high potential for painful consequences
Bipolar II disorder	≥4 days *AND*	Hypomania: abnormally, persistently elevated or irritable mood; persistently increased energy or activity *without* psychosis or hospitalization

TABLE 8–1. Abbreviated DSM-5-TR criteria for common diagnoses *(continued)*

Diagnosis	Criteria/time	Symptoms
	≥3	Inflated self-esteem or grandiosity; decreased need for sleep; pressured speech; flight of ideas or racing thoughts; distractibility; increased goal-directed activity; excessive involvement in activities with high potential for painful consequences
Depressive disorders		
Disruptive mood dysregulation disorder	≥3 outbursts per week for ≥12 months	Severe recurrent temper outbursts manifested verbally and/or behaviorally that are out of proportion to the situation and inconsistent with developmental level (diagnosis cannot be made in children younger than 6 years)
		Mood between outbursts is persistently irritable or angry most of the day, nearly every day, and observable by others
Major depressive disorder	≥1 for ≥2 weeks *AND*	Depressed mood; marked loss of interest in activities or pleasure (anhedonia)
	≥4 for ≥2 weeks	Significant unintentional weight loss or decreased appetite; insomnia or hypersomnia; psychomotor agitation or retardation; fatigue or loss of energy; worthlessness or excessive guilt; decreased ability to concentrate; recurrent thoughts of death or suicide

TABLE 8–1. Abbreviated DSM-5-TR criteria for common diagnoses *(continued)*

Diagnosis	Criteria/time	Symptoms
Anxiety disorders		
Separation anxiety disorder	≥3 for ≥4 weeks	Excessive distress with separation from home or caregivers; persistent worry about harm to caregivers; excessive worry about untoward event separating from caregiver; excessive reluctance to be alone; persistent reluctance to sleep away from home; repetitive nightmares about separation; repeated physical symptoms when separating
Panic disorder	≥4 *AND*	Recurrent surges of intense fear or intense discomfort demonstrated by palpitations; sweating; trembling; shortness of breath; choking sensation; chest pain; nausea; dizziness; chills; paresthesias; derealization; fear of losing control or becoming insane; fear of death
	≥1 month	Persistent concern or worry about panic attacks *OR* Maladaptive change in behavior related to attacks
Generalized anxiety disorder	≥3 *AND*	Restlessness; easily fatigued; difficulty concentrating; irritability; muscle tension; sleep disturbance

TABLE 8–1. Abbreviated DSM-5-TR criteria for common diagnoses (*continued*)

Diagnosis	Criteria/time	Symptoms
	≥6 months	Excessive anxiety and worry (apprehensive expectation) that is difficult to control
Obsessive-compulsive and related disorders		
OCD	≥1 hour/day	Obsessions: recurrent and intrusive thoughts, urges, images that a person attempts to ignore or suppress through compulsive acts *AND/OR* Compulsions: repetitive behaviors or mental acts to reduce distress
Trauma- and stressor-related disorders		
Reactive attachment disorder	Both beginning before 5 years old	Experience of extreme insufficient care Consistent pattern of emotionally withdrawn behavior toward caregivers; persistent social and emotional disturbance
PTSD (6 years or younger)	*AND*	Exposure to actual or threatened death, serious injury, or sexual violence, especially of primary caregivers
	≥1 for ≥1 month *AND*	Intrusions: distressing memories, which may be reenacted in play; intrusive dreams; dissociative flashbacks; exposures to triggers causing intense or prolonged distress; marked physiological reactions

Common DSM-5-TR Diagnoses   **201**

TABLE 8–1. Abbreviated DSM-5-TR criteria for common diagnoses (*continued*)

Diagnosis	Criteria/time	Symptoms
Trauma- and stressor-related disorders (*continued*)		
PTSD (6 years or younger) (*continued*)	≥1 for ≥1 month *AND* ≥2 for ≥1 month *AND*	Avoidance: internal reminders; external reminders of trauma
		Negative symptom: impaired memory of trauma; negative self-worth; pathological blame; negative emotional states; decreased participation; detachment; emotional numbness
	≥2 for ≥1 month	Reactive arousal: irritability or aggression, including extreme temper tantrums; recklessness; hypervigilance; exaggerated startle response; impaired concentration; sleep disturbance
PTSD (older than 6 years)	*AND*	Exposure to actual or threatened death, serious injury, or sexual violence
	≥1 for ≥1 month *AND*	Intrusions: distressing memories; intrusive dreams; flashbacks; exposures to triggers causing distress; marked physiological reactions
	≥1 for ≥1 month *AND*	Avoidance: internal reminders; external reminders of trauma

TABLE 8–1. Abbreviated DSM-5-TR criteria for common diagnoses *(continued)*

Diagnosis	Criteria/time	Symptoms
	≥2 for ≥1 month *AND*	Negative symptom: impaired memory of trauma; negative self-worth; pathological blame; negative emotional states; decreased participation; detachment; emotional numbness
	≥2 for ≥1 month	Reactive arousal: irritability or aggression, including extreme temper tantrums; recklessness; hypervigilance; exaggerated startle response; impaired concentration; sleep disturbance
Feeding and eating disorders		
Pica	≥1 month	Persistent consumption of nonnutritive, nonfood substances that is inconsistent with developmental stage and cultural practices
Anorexia nervosa	All 3	Persistent energy intake restriction; intense fear of gaining weight or persistent behavior that interferes with weight gain; disturbance in self-perceived body shape or weight
Bulimia nervosa	Both at least weekly for ≥3 months	Recurrent episodes of binge eating; self-evaluation unduly influenced by body shape and weight
		Recurrent inappropriate compensatory behaviors to prevent weight gain

TABLE 8–1. Abbreviated DSM-5-TR criteria for common diagnoses (*continued*)

Diagnosis	Criteria/time	Symptoms
Elimination disorders		
Enuresis (≥5 years)	≥2 times weekly for ≥3 months	Repeated passage of urine into bed or clothes not attributable to a substance or another medical condition
Encopresis (≥4 years)	≥1 monthly for ≥3 months	Repeated passage of feces into inappropriate places not attributable to a substance or another medical condition
Disruptive, impulse-control, and conduct disorders		
Oppositional defiant disorder	≥4 for ≥6 months; if younger than 5 years, symptoms on most days; if older than 5 years, symptoms at least weekly	Often loses temper; often touchy or easily annoyed; often angry and resentful; often argues with adults; often defies rules or authority figures; often annoys others; often blames others; spiteful or vindictive
Intermittent explosive disorder	≥1 in a person ≥6 years	Recurrent, impulsive (or anger-based) verbal outbursts ≥2 times weekly for ≥3 months; ≥3 impulsive (or anger-based) behavioral outbursts resulting in property damage or injury to animals or persons in a 12-month period

TABLE 8–1. Abbreviated DSM-5-TR criteria for common diagnoses *(continued)*

Diagnosis	Criteria/time	Symptoms
Conduct disorder	≥3 in the past 12 months *AND* ≥1 in the past 6 months	Often bullies or threatens others; often initiates physical fights; uses a weapon; physically cruel to people; physically cruel to animals; stealing while confronting a victim; forcing someone into sexual activity; deliberately sets fire to cause damage; deliberately destroys property; breaks into someone else's dwelling or car; frequently lies to obtain favors or avoid obligations; steals items of nontrivial value; stays out at night without permission; runs away from home overnight; often truant from school

Source. American Psychiatric Association 2022.

Chapter 9

Taking Six Steps to a Differential Diagnosis

Because a person's mental distress can be explained in multiple ways, a good clinician considers many diagnoses when pursuing their explanation of a patient's distress (Feinstein 1967). As a clinician develops their clinical decision-making, it is helpful to investigate different explanatory possibilities sequentially to develop their habit of reflecting on what psychiatrist Kenneth Kendler (2012, p. 377) called "the dappled nature," the many and interrelated causes, of mental disorders. Clinicians interested in exploring further steps in differential diagnosis should read texts specific to psychiatric evaluation (e.g., Chisolm and Lyketsos 2012) and the *DSM-5-TR Handbook of Differential Diagnosis* (First 2022).

Step 1: Could the Signs and Symptoms Be Intentionally Produced?

Consider whether a patient might be intentionally producing findings, because an honest report of psychiatric symptoms and signs is the foundation for developing a fruitful diagnosis and treatment plan. An honest report strengthens the therapeutic alliance, just as a dishonest report weakens the therapeutic alliance. If intentionally produced findings are associated with an obvious external award—such as time off from school or family activity or a change in caregivers—consider the possibility of malingering. Malingering may be concomitant with other medical and psychiatric diagnoses. If intentionally produced findings are associated with the desire to be perceived as ill or impaired, consider factitious disorder.

A patient can also unconsciously produce signs or symptoms to resolve a psychological conflict, to validate their inability to function socially, or as an attempt to secure assistance. In these situations, consider one of the somatic symptom and related disorders.

Step 2: Are the Signs and Symptoms Related to a Developmental Stage or Conflict?

If you are thoroughly evaluating a young child, your evaluation should eventually include a developmental assessment. Even when you are interviewing older children, adolescents, and adults, however, you should consider a patient's developmental stage, which can be quite different from the developmental stage you would expect on the basis of their age, background, and education (summarized in Chapter 13, "Recognizing Developmental Red Flags"). A thorough social history also will give you a sense of how a patient's current behavior relates to their usual behavior. Even in a brief interview, it is useful to observe how your patient communicates and behaves and compare their communication and behavior with those appropriate for their age, culture, and education. If you observe a disjunction, consider these possibilities:

- The patient is experiencing a transient regression in response to a particular event.
- The patient is using an immature defense mechanism, which may indicate a personality trait or disorder.
- The patient is experiencing a developmental conflict in a particular relationship.
- The patient has a developmental delay or intellectual impairment.

Step 3: Are the Signs and Symptoms Related to a Caregiver Conflict?

Human beings are, in the words of the philosopher Alasdair MacIntyre, "dependent rational animals" because we depend on "particular others for protection and sustenance" (MacIntyre 2012, p. 1). This dependence is acute for children and adolescents. By degrees of ability, age, development, impairment, and temperament, children and adolescents depend on both adults and fellow children as caregivers. Caregivers can aid or injure a child or an adolescent. As you evaluate a child or an adolescent, observe how they do (or do not) speak about the caregivers in their life, either directly or through transitional objects. As you observe, consider these possibilities:

- A caregiver and the patient have communication difficulties or cultural differences.
- A caregiver is a poor fit with the patient.
- A caregiver is abusing, neglecting, or otherwise harming the patient.

Step 4: Are the Signs and Symptoms Related to Substances?

People use and misuse a variety of substances, which results in varied clinical effects. People can experience mental distress during substance use, intoxication, and withdrawal. When you seek the cause of a patient's distress, always consider drugs of abuse, as well as prescription, over-the-counter, and herbal medicines or products. People often underreport their use of substances, so consider these possibilities:

- Substances may directly cause a patient's psychiatric signs and symptoms.
- A patient may use substances because of a mental disorder and its sequelae.
- A patient may use substances and experience psychiatric signs and symptoms, but the substance use and the signs and symptoms are unrelated.

Step 5: Are the Signs and Symptoms Related to Another Medical Condition?

A patient can present with another medical condition that mimics psychiatric signs and symptoms. Sometimes, presentation with these findings is a sentinel event that occurs in advance of the other stigmata of a medical condition. Alternatively, a patient may develop psychiatric signs and symptoms years after their presentation for another medical condition. Clues that another medical condition may be related to a mental disorder include an atypical presentation, atypical age at onset, and atypical course. Consider these possibilities:

- Another medical condition directly alters the patient's psychiatric signs and symptoms.
- Another medical condition indirectly alters the patient's psychiatric signs and symptoms, as through a psychological mechanism.
- The treatment for another medical condition directly alters the patient's psychiatric signs and symptoms.
- The patient's mental disorder, or its treatment, causes or exacerbates another medical condition.
- The patient has a mental disorder and another medical condition, but they are causally unrelated.

Step 6: To What Extent Are the Signs and Symptoms Related to a Mental Disorder?

DSM-5-TR (American Psychiatric Association 2022) diagnoses are summaries of information that allow you to categorize the experiences of a distressed child or adolescent and to communicate with the other professionals caring for that patient. A good clinician relies on the predominant symptomatology to support their diagnosis. DSM-5-TR seeks parsimony, but diagnoses are not mutually exclusive, so consider these possibilities:

- Condition A may predispose a patient to Condition B and vice versa.
- An underlying condition, such as a genetic predisposition, may make a patient susceptible to both Conditions A and B.
- A mediating factor, such as alterations in reward systems, may influence susceptibility to both Conditions A and B.
- Conditions A and B may be part of a more complex and unified syndrome that has been artificially split in the diagnostic system.
- The relationship between Conditions A and B may be artificially enhanced by overlaps in the diagnostic criteria.
- The comorbidity between Conditions A and B may be coincidental.

A Final Thought: Could It Be That No Mental Disorder Is Present?

After working toward a diagnosis, it helps to take a step back and remember: "normality" covers a wide range of behaviors and thoughts that vary across cultural groups and developmental stages. According to DSM-5-TR, a mental disorder causes a "clinically significant disturbance in an individual's cognition, emotion regulation, or behavior that reflects a dysfunction in the psychological, biological, or developmental processes underlying mental functioning" (American Psychiatric Association 2022, p. 14). When a patient's symptoms and presentation cause clinically significant distress or impairment without fulfilling the criteria for a specific mental disorder, consider the following alternatives:

- An *other specified* diagnosis, in which a practitioner specifies why a patient's experience does not meet the criteria for a specific diagnosis.
- An *unspecified* diagnosis, in which a practitioner does not specify why a patient's experience does not meet the criteria for a specific diagnosis. (This diagnosis implies that you presently have insufficient information to make an other specified diagnosis.)
- No psychiatric diagnosis at all. Many people live with one, two, or even several signs or symptoms of mental illness without those symptoms meeting criteria for any DSM-5-TR mental disorder. After all, the boundaries between normality and abnormality are determined through the exercise of a clinician's experienced judgment and a culture's shifting sanctions.

Chapter 10

Organizing a Comprehensive Pediatric Mental Status Examination With a Psychiatric Glossary

A comprehensive pediatric mental status examination begins with a patient's outer appearance and progressively proceeds into their interior life. To make the journey from appearance to insight, a clinician carefully observes and thoughtfully questions a patient, all while keeping in mind cultural context, developmental stage, and education level. To describe their findings, clinicians use a specialized language that can be learned from psychiatric glossaries (see Shahrokh et al. 2011 and the appendix to DSM-5-TR [American Psychiatric Association 2022]). A clinician can organize their experience of a patient's mental state using their own version of the format outlined here, which includes definitions for the essential terms for the mental status examination.

Appearance

Describe how the patient appears, which may include the following:

- Ability to make and maintain eye contact
- Appropriateness to the situation
- Attitude toward the interview
- Cleanliness
- Dress
- Grooming
- Habitus (general constitution and physical build)
- Posture

Behavior

Document the patient's behaviors, which may include the following:

- Ability to relate socially during your encounter
- Ability to enact play, both individually and with others
- Ambulatory status and, if possible, gait
- Catalepsy (maintenance of any physical position after being moved by examiner)
- Posturing (striking a pose and maintaining it)
- Drooling
- Mannerisms (unnecessary behaviors that are part of goal-directed behavior)
- Presence of waxy flexibility (resistance of limbs to passive motion that improves with ongoing movement)
- Psychomotor agitation (excessive physical activity accompanied by inner tension)
- Psychomotor retardation (generalized slowing of cognitive, emotional, or physical responses)
- Stereotypies (non-goal-directed behaviors that are unusual in frequency but not in the action itself)
- Signs of extrapyramidal symptoms or tardive dyskinesia
- Tics (involuntary, recurrent, nonrhythmic movement or vocalization)
- Tremor

Speech and Language

Describe or note (if present) the following characteristics of the patient's speech:

- Amount
- Latency (a pause of several seconds before responding to a question)
- Rate
- Rhythm
- Tone
- Volume

Document the following speech problems, if present:

- Anomia (inability to name everyday objects)
- Dysnomia (inability to find words)

Emotion

Describe, if present, the following characteristics of the patient's emotional state:

- Affect (the emotional tone conveyed by speech and behaviors)
- Alexithymia (inability to describe or recognize one's own emotions)
- Appropriateness to the situation
- Intensity
- Mood (the emotional state that is sustained throughout the encounter)
- Quality
- Range
- Stability

Thought Process

Describe how the patient thinks, and note any evidence of the following:

- Mutism (absence of speech)
- Alliteration
- Aphonia (ability to only whisper or croak)
- Clang association (words chosen purely for sound)
- Decreased latency of response (answering questions before you can finish asking them)
- Increased latency of response (long pauses before fairly normal speech)
- Derailment (running ideas into each other)
- Distractibility (being easily diverted by extraneous stimuli)
- Echolalia (repetition of words or statements of others)
- Flight of ideas (an illogical group of associations)
- Associations may be described as intact, circumstantial (providing unnecessary details but eventually answering a question), tangential (only initially responding to a question), loose (providing responses unrelated to a question), or even word salad (random use of words)
- Neologisms (creation of words)
- Perseveration (repetition of the same motor or verbal response despite varied stimuli)

- Poverty of speech (brief, concrete responses with limited spontaneous speech)
- Push of speech (increased, rapid speech that is often loud and difficult to interrupt)
- Verbigeration (prolonged repetition of isolated words)

Thought Content

Comment on what the person discusses, including the presence of any of the following:

- Compulsions (irresistible impulses to perform a behavior)
- Obsessions (recurrent, persistent ideas, images, or desires that dominate thought)
- Delusions (fixed, firm, false beliefs that are not part of the person's culture or religion)
- Grandiosity
- Guilt
- Hallucinations (perceptions of an absent stimulus)
- Illusions (misperceptions of an actual stimulus)
- Ideas of persecution
- Ideas of reference (perceptions that unrelated stimuli have a particular and unusual meaning specific to the person)
- Ideation, intent, or plan to harm self or others (suicidal, homicidal, or violent)
- Paranoia
- Passivity (submissive attitude toward a perceived superior)
- Phobias (intense, unreasonable, specific fears)
- Thought insertion (the perception that one's thoughts are not one's own but are inserted into one's mind by others)
- Thought withdrawal (the perception that others can take thoughts out of one's mind without consent)

Cognition

Observe and comment on the patient's cognition and intellectual resources related to their developmental age, including the following:

- Ability to abstract and to interpret culturally and educationally appropriate proverbs

- Ability to calculate
- Ability to read and write
- Fund of general information
- Learning style
- Impulse control
- Orientation
- Recent and remote memory
- When known, comment on the person's IQ and learning style.

Insight and Judgment

Observe and comment on the patient's insight and judgment, including the following:

- Insight into their condition, especially as to whether they deny or appreciate their problem
- Judgment (mental ability to compare choices and make appropriate decisions) as related to the presenting condition and age

PART III

Additional Tools and Clinical Guidance

Chapter 11

Using DSM-5-TR Assessment Measures to Aid Diagnosis

The authors of DSM-5-TR (American Psychiatric Association 2022) describe the manual as subject to revision as the science underlying psychiatry advances. They even hint at the manual's eventual successors in Section III, "Emerging Measures and Models," which includes several assessment tools, rating scales, and alternative diagnoses. Taken together, these constitute valuable tools for current use and ways forward for DSM as a diagnostic system.

At present, the main text of DSM-5-TR preserves the categorical model of mental illness. The categorical model, in which a person does or does not have a mental illness on the basis of the presence or absence of symptoms, was first introduced in DSM-III (American Psychiatric Association 1980). The categorical model holds together the various clinicians and researchers who care for and study persons with mental illness by giving them a shared text, even though they may favor different accounts of mental illness, for current clinical work (Kinghorn 2011).

The great achievement of the categorical model has been increased diagnostic reliability (i.e., the ability of different clinicians to agree on the same diagnosis for a particular person). The great shortcoming of the categorical model has been limited diagnostic validity (i.e., the ability of clinicians to make an accurate diagnosis) (Kendell and Jablensky 2003).

In various ways, each of the tools in Section III of DSM-5-TR attempts to improve the reliability and validity of psychiatric diagnoses. These tools are diverse, but we find that all these measures can be used by clinicians to personalize the diagnostic criteria for a particular patient. In this chapter, we introduce several of these measures as aids to clinical practice with children and adolescents.

Level 1 and 2 Cross-Cutting Symptom Measures

Most young people first seek help for mental distress from someone they already know. Within medicine, this is usually a physician, nurse, school counselor, or other professional whose principal role or specialty is not the provision of mental health services. Indeed, most mental health care occurs in the offices of primary care clinicians. To address the gap between the mental health training these clinicians possess and the volume of mental health care they provide, DSM-5-TR provides screening tools for use in either primary care or mental health settings. These brief, plain-language tools can be completed before a clinical encounter by the patient or someone who knows them well. The tools are available in this chapter, in Section III of DSM-5-TR, and online at www.psychiatry.org/dsm5. They can be reproduced and used, without additional permission, for clinical and research evaluations.

Each tool has a series of short questions about recent symptoms; for example, "During the past two (2) weeks, how much (or how often) has your child seemed angry or lost his/her temper?" These screening questions assess core symptoms for the major diagnoses. For each symptom statement, a patient or their caregiver assesses how much this bothered the patient on a 5-point scale: none (0), slight (1), mild (2), moderate (3), or severe (4). Each tool is designed to be easily scored. If a patient reports a clinically significant problem in any domain, you should consider using a more detailed assessment tool; in this example, that would be a tool for assessing anger.

DSM-5-TR includes a hierarchy of screening tools. The initial assessment, described in the previous paragraph, is the Level 1 Cross-Cutting Symptom Measure, which is completed before an initial evaluation by the person seeking assessment or by the caregiver of a child or an adolescent. The version for children ages 6–17 (there is no version for children younger than 6) includes 25 questions assessing 12 domains and is available in a format for a child or an adolescent to complete on their own or for a caregiver to complete. For most, but not all, of the symptom domains screened for in the Level 1 Cross-Cutting Symptom Measure, separate Level 2 Cross-Cutting Symptom Measures are available for specific areas of concern, including anger, anxiety, depression, inattention, mania, repetitive thoughts and behaviors, sleep disturbance, somatic symptom, and substance use.

When Level 1 and 2 assessments are used, they can help a clinician identify and characterize the presenting problems. But they have another potential benefit after the initial assessment: helping to measure treatment response and progress toward recovery. DSM-5-TR suggests using the Level 2 Cross-Cutting Symptom Measures at your first evaluation of a patient in part so that you can establish a baseline and then revisit that assessment periodically to assess progress. These measures assess dimensions rather than diagnoses, which means they are not designed to tell you the degree of likelihood of identifying a specific diagnosis. Their strength is that they allow you to track different symptom domains, such as the depressive symptoms of a patient with schizophrenia in addition to their psychotic symptoms.

Systematic use of these cross-cutting assessments alerts you to significant changes in a patient's symptomatology and provides measurable outcomes for treatment plans. The assessments alert researchers to lacunae in the current diagnostic system. For your convenience, Figures 11–1 and 11–2 show the child- and caregiver-rated versions of the Level 1 tool.

Practitioners using the Level 1 tools are encouraged to further explore reports of even seemingly slight problems with inattention, psychosis, substance use, and suicidal ideation or attempts. For the other domains, practitioners are encouraged to explore symptoms identified at the next higher level of severity (mild or several days) or greater. The Level 2 measures are easily accessed online at www.psychiatry.org/psychiatrists/practice/dsm/educational-resources/assessment-measures. The suggested Level 2 measures are described in Table 11–1.

Cultural Formulation Interview

The authors of DSM-5 (American Psychiatric Association 2013) are improving the diagnostic system by attending to the cultural specificity of mental distress and illness. Asking about a patient's and caregiver's cultural understanding of sickness and health is an efficient way to build a therapeutic alliance while gathering pertinent information (Lim 2015). In addition, performing a cultural assessment personalizes the diagnosis, which increases its accuracy (Bäärnhielm and Scarpinati

Name: _____   Age: _____   Sex: ☐ Male ☐ Female   Date: _____

Instructions: The questions below ask about things that might have bothered you. For each question, circle the number that best describes how much (or how often) you have been bothered by each problem during the **past TWO (2) WEEKS.**

	During the past **TWO (2) WEEKS,** how much (or how often) have you...	None Not at all	Slight Rare, less than a day or two	Mild Several days	Moderate More than half the days	Severe Nearly every day	Highest Domain Score (clinician)
I.	1. Been bothered by stomachaches, headaches, or other aches and pains?	0	1	2	3	4	
	2. Worried about your health or about getting sick?	0	1	2	3	4	
II.	3. Been bothered by not being able to fall asleep or stay asleep, or by waking up too early?	0	1	2	3	4	
III.	4. Been bothered by not being able to pay attention when you were in class or doing homework or reading a book or playing a game?	0	1	2	3	4	
IV.	5. Had less fun doing things than you used to?	0	1	2	3	4	
	6. Felt sad or depressed for several hours?	0	1	2	3	4	
V. &	7. Felt more irritated or easily annoyed than usual?	0	1	2	3	4	
VI.	8. Felt angry or lost your temper?	0	1	2	3	4	

FIGURE 11–1. DSM-5-TR Self-Rated Level 1 Cross-Cutting Symptom Measure—Child Age 11–17.

		None Not at all	Slight Rare, less than a day or two	Mild Several days	Moderate More than half the days	Severe Nearly every day	Highest Domain Score (clinician)
	During the past TWO (2) WEEKS, how much (or how often) have you...						
VII.	9. Started lots more projects than usual or done more risky things than usual?	0	1	2	3	4	
	10. Slept less than usual but still had a lot of energy?	0	1	2	3	4	
VIII.	11. Felt nervous, anxious, or scared?	0	1	2	3	4	
	12. Not been able to stop worrying?	0	1	2	3	4	
	13. Not been able to do things you wanted to or should have done, because they made you feel nervous?	0	1	2	3	4	
IX.	14. Heard voices—when there was no one there—speaking about you or telling you what to do or saying bad things to you?	0	1	2	3	4	
	15. Had visions when you were completely awake—that is, seen something or someone that no one else could see?	0	1	2	3	4	

FIGURE 11–1. DSM-5-TR Self-Rated Level 1 Cross-Cutting Symptom Measure—Child Age 11–17. *(continued)*

During the past **TWO (2) WEEKS**, how much (or how often) have you...	None Not at all	Slight Rare, less than a day or two	Mild Several days	Moderate More than half the days	Severe Nearly every day	Highest Domain Score (clinician)
X.						
16. Had thoughts that kept coming into your mind that you would do something bad or that something bad would happen to you or to someone else?	0	1	2	3	4	
17. Felt the need to check on certain things over and over again, like whether a door was locked or whether the stove was turned off?	0	1	2	3	4	
18. Worried a lot about things you touched being dirty or having germs or being poisoned?	0	1	2	3	4	
19. Felt you had to do things in a certain way, like counting or saying special things, to keep something bad from happening?	0	1	2	3	4	

FIGURE 11–1. DSM-5-TR Self-Rated Level 1 Cross-Cutting Symptom Measure—Child Age 11–17. (*continued*)

		In the past **TWO (2) WEEKS,** have you...		
XI.	20.	Had an alcoholic beverage (beer, wine, liquor, etc.)?	☐ Yes	☐ No
	21.	Smoked a cigarette, a cigar, or pipe, or used snuff or chewing tobacco?	☐ Yes	☐ No
	22.	Used drugs like marijuana, cocaine or crack, club drugs (like Ecstasy), hallucinogens (like LSD), heroin, inhalants or solvents (like glue), or methamphetamine (like speed)?	☐ Yes	☐ No
	23.	Used any medicine without a doctor's prescription to get high or change the way you feel (e.g., painkillers [like Vicodin], stimulants [like Ritalin or Adderall], sedatives or tranquilizers [like sleeping pills or Valium], or steroids)?	☐ Yes	☐ No
XII.	24.	In the last 2 weeks, have you thought about killing yourself or committing suicide?	☐ Yes	☐ No
	25.	Have you EVER tried to kill yourself?	☐ Yes	☐ No

FIGURE 11–1. DSM-5-TR Self-Rated Level 1 Cross-Cutting Symptom Measure—Child Age 11–17. *(continued)*

Child's Name: _____   Age: _____   Sex: ☐ Male ☐ Female   Date: _____

Relationship with the child: _____

Instructions *(to the parent or guardian of child)*: The questions below ask about things that might have bothered your child. For each question, circle the number that best describes how much (or how often) your child has been bothered by each problem during the past **TWO (2) WEEKS.**

	During the past **TWO (2) WEEKS**, how much (or how often) has your child...	**None** Not at all	**Slight** Rare, less than a day or two	**Mild** Several days	**Moderate** More than half the days	**Severe** Nearly every day	**Highest Domain Score** (clinician)
I.	1. Complained of stomachaches, headaches, or other aches and pains?	0	1	2	3	4	
	2. Said he/she was worried about his/her health or about getting sick?	0	1	2	3	4	
II.	3. Had problems sleeping—that is, trouble falling asleep, staying asleep, or waking up too early?	0	1	2	3	4	
III.	4. Had problems paying attention when he/she was in class or doing his/her homework or reading a book or playing a game?	0	1	2	3	4	
IV.	5. Had less fun doing things than he/she used to?	0	1	2	3	4	
	6. Seemed sad or depressed for several hours?	0	1	2	3	4	

FIGURE 11–2. DSM-5-TR Parent/Guardian-Rated DSM-5 Level 1 Cross-Cutting Symptom Measure—Child Age 6–17.

			None Not at all	Slight Rare, less than a day or two	Mild Several days	Moderate More than half the days	Severe Nearly every day	Highest Domain Score (clinician)
		During the past **TWO (2) WEEKS**, how much (or how often) has your child...						
V. &	7.	Seemed more irritated or easily annoyed than usual?	0	1	2	3	4	
VI.	8.	Seemed angry or lost his/her temper?	0	1	2	3	4	
VII.	9.	Started lots more projects than usual or did more risky things than usual?	0	1	2	3	4	
	10.	Slept less than usual for him/her, but still had lots of energy?	0	1	2	3	4	
VIII.	11.	Said he/she felt nervous, anxious, or scared?	0	1	2	3	4	
	12.	Not been able to stop worrying?	0	1	2	3	4	
	13.	Said he/she couldn't do things he/she wanted to or should have done, because they made him/her feel nervous?	0	1	2	3	4	
IX.	14.	Said that he/she heard voices—when there was no one there—speaking about him/her or telling him/her what to do or saying bad things to him/her?	0	1	2	3	4	
	15.	Said that he/she had a vision when he/she was completely awake—that is, saw something or someone that no one else could see?	0	1	2	3	4	

FIGURE 11–2. DSM-5-TR Parent/Guardian-Rated DSM-5 Level 1 Cross-Cutting Symptom Measure—Child Age 6–17. *(continued)*

	During the past **TWO (2) WEEKS,** how much (or how often) has your child...	**None** Not at all	**Slight** Rare, less than a day or two	**Mild** Several days	**Moderate** More than half the days	**Severe** Nearly every day	**Highest Domain Score** (clinician)
X.							
16.	Said that he/she had thoughts that kept coming into his/her mind that he/she would do something bad or that something bad would happen to him/her or to someone else?	0	1	2	3	4	
17.	Said he/she felt the need to check on certain things over and over again, like whether a door was locked or whether the stove was turned off?	0	1	2	3	4	
18.	Seemed to worry a lot about things he/she touched being dirty or having germs or being poisoned?	0	1	2	3	4	
19.	Said that he/she had to do things in a certain way, like counting or saying special things out loud, in order to keep something bad from happening?	0	1	2	3	4	

FIGURE 11–2. DSM-5-TR Parent/Guardian-Rated DSM-5 Level 1 Cross-Cutting Symptom Measure—Child Age 6–17. *(continued)*

	In the past **TWO (2) WEEKS,** has your child ...				
XI.	20. Had an alcoholic beverage (beer, wine, liquor, etc.)?	☐ Yes	☐ No	☐ Don't Know	
	21. Smoked a cigarette, a cigar, or pipe, or used snuff or chewing tobacco?	☐ Yes	☐ No	☐ Don't Know	
	22. Used drugs like marijuana, cocaine or crack, club drugs (like ecstasy), hallucinogens (like LSD), heroin, inhalants or solvents (like glue), or methamphetamine (like speed)?	☐ Yes	☐ No	☐ Don't Know	
	23. Used any medicine without a doctor's prescription (e.g., painkillers [like Vicodin], stimulants [like Ritalin or Adderall], sedatives or tranquilizers [like sleeping pills or Valium], or steroids)?	☐ Yes	☐ No	☐ Don't Know	
XII.	24. In the past **TWO (2) WEEKS,** has he/she talked about wanting to kill himself/herself or about wanting to commit suicide?	☐ Yes	☐ No	☐ Don't Know	
	25. Has he/she EVER tried to kill himself/herself?	☐ Yes	☐ No	☐ Don't Know	

FIGURE 11–2. DSM-5-TR Parent/Guardian-Rated DSM-5 Level 1 Cross-Cutting Symptom Measure—Child Age 6–17. (*continued*)

TABLE 11–1. Parent/guardian-rated DSM-5-TR Level 1 Cross-Cutting Symptom Measure for Child Age 6–17: 12 domains, thresholds for further inquiry, and associated Level 2 measures

Domain	Domain name	Threshold to guide further inquiry	DSM-5-TR Level 2 Cross-Cutting Symptom Measure[a]
I.	Somatic symptoms	Mild or greater	Level 2—Somatic Symptom—Child Age 11–17 (Patient Health Questionnaire–15 [PHQ-15] Somatic Symptom Severity Scale)
II.	Sleep problems	Mild or greater	Level 2—Sleep Disturbance—Child Age 11–17 (PROMIS—Sleep Disturbance—Short Form)
III.	Inattention	Slight or greater	Level 2—Inattention—Parent/Guardian of Child Age 6–17 (Swanson, Nolan, and Pelham, Version IV [SNAP-IV])
IV.	Depression	Mild or greater	Level 2—Depression—Parent/Guardian of Child Age 11–17 (PROMIS Emotional Distress—Depression—Parent Item Bank)
V.	Anger	Mild or greater	Level 2—Anger—Parent/Guardian of Child (PROMIS Calibrated Anger Measure—Parent)
VI.	Irritability	Mild or greater	Level 2—Irritability—Parent/Guardian of Child (Affective Reactivity Index [ARI])

TABLE 11–1. Parent/guardian-rated DSM-5-TR Level 1 Cross-Cutting Symptom Measure for Child Age 6–17: 12 domains, thresholds for further inquiry, and associated Level 2 measures (continued)

Domain	Domain name	Threshold to guide further inquiry	DSM-5-TR Level 2 Cross-Cutting Symptom Measure[a]
VII.	Mania	Mild or greater	Level 2—Mania—Parent/Guardian of Child Age 11–17 (Altman Self-Rating Mania Scale [ASRM])
VIII.	Anxiety	Mild or greater	Level 2—Anxiety—Parent/Guardian of Child Age 11–17 (PROMIS Emotional Distress—Anxiety—Parent Item Bank)
IX.	Psychosis	Slight or greater	None
X.	Repetitive thoughts and behaviors	Mild or greater	None
XI.	Substance use	Yes/Don't know	Level 2—Substance Use—Parent/Guardian of Child Age 11–17 (adapted from the NIDA-modified ASSIST)
XII.	Suicidal ideation/ suicide attempts	Yes/Don't know	None

Note.   NIDA=National Institute on Drug Abuse.

[a]Available online at www.psychiatry.org/psychiatrists/practice/dsm/educational-resources/assessment-measures.

Rosso 2009). In Section III of DSM-5-TR, in "Cultural Concepts of Distress," the authors discuss cultural syndromes, cultural idioms of distress, and cultural explanations of perceived causes.

To use this cultural information in a diagnostic interview, it is beneficial to first define three types of cultural concepts. A *cultural syndrome* is a group of clustered psychiatric symptoms specific to a particular culture or community. The syndrome provides a coherent pattern for experiences. A classic example is *ataque de nervios*, a syndrome of mental distress characterized by the sudden onset of intense fear, often experienced physically as a sensation of heat rising in the chest, which may result in aggressive or suicidal behavior (Lewis-Fernández et al. 2016). The syndrome is often associated with familial distress in Latino communities across DSM-5-TR diagnostic categories (Lizardi et al. 2009). A *cultural idiom of distress* is a collective, shared way of expressing distress outside of a specific syndrome or symptom, say, "nerves" instead of *ataque de nervios* or generalized anxiety disorder. Finally, a *cultural explanation of perceived cause* provides an explanatory model of why mental distress or illness occurs, and the cultural explanation can be folk or professional, because both indigenous communities and medical societies constitute a culture (American Psychiatric Association 2022).

The Cultural Formulation Interview (CFI) is a semistructured tool, updated for DSM-5-TR, for assessing the influence of culture in a particular patient's experience of distress. The CFI can be used at any time during a diagnostic interview, especially when you struggle to reach a diagnosis because of cultural differences between you and a patient, when you are uncertain whether diagnostic criteria map onto a cultural concept, when you are laboring to assess the dimensional severity of a diagnosis, when you and a patient have divergent understandings of treatment, when you and a patient disagree on treatment, when a patient may mistrust health services because of a collective traumatic experience, or when a patient is disengaged during an interview (American Psychiatric Association 2022).

Over the past decade, the use of the CFI has been studied in Canada, Kenya, Mexico, the Netherlands, Peru, and the United States (Jarvis et al. 2020). Researchers have found that undertaking even a single hour of CFI training can increase a clinician's cultural competence (Mills et al. 2016), and CFI training can be delivered through online curricula (Aggarwal et al. 2018). The CFI can be the foundation of a culturally competent clinical service (Díaz et al. 2017).

You should not limit use of the CFI to situations in which you perceive the patient as being culturally different from yourself. You can use the CFI in any setting because "cultural" accounts of why people get ill and why people return to health occur in all communities. People with whom you believe you share a cultural account of illness and health often have a very different understanding of why people become ill and how they can become well. Finally, the CFI is the most patient-centered portion of DSM-5-TR, and using it particularizes the diagnostic process. The CFI is not a scored system of symptoms but rather a series of prompts to help you assess how a patient understands their distress, its etiology, its treatment, and their prognosis. Online, at www.psychiatry.org/dsm5, you can find alternative versions of the CFI and supplementary modules. Here, we include an adapted version of the supplemental CFI questions specific to children and adolescents.

Suggested introduction to the child or adolescent: *We have talked about the concerns of your family. Now I would like to know more about how you feel about being ___ years old.*

Feelings of age appropriateness in different settings: *Do you feel you are like other people your age? In what way? Do you sometimes feel different from other people your age? In what way?*

If the child or adolescent acknowledges sometimes feeling different: *Does this feeling of being different happen more at home, at school, at work, and/or in some other place? Do you feel that your family is different from other families? Do you use different languages? With whom and when? Does your name have any special meaning for you? Your family? Your community? Is there something special about you that you like or that you are proud of?*

Age-related stressors and supports: *What do you like about being a person at home? At school? With friends? What don't you like about being a person at home? At school? With friends? Who is there to support you when you feel you need it? At home? At school? Among your friends?*

Age-related expectations: *What do your parents or grandparents expect from a person your age in terms of chores, schoolwork, play, or religious observance? What do your schoolteachers expect from a person your age?*

If the child or adolescent has siblings: *What do your siblings expect from a person your age? What do other people your age expect from a person your age?*

Transition to adulthood/maturity (for adolescents only):
Are there any important celebrations or events in your community to recognize reaching a certain age or growing up? When is a youth considered ready to become an adult in your family or community? When is a youth considered ready to become an adult according to your schoolteachers? What is good or difficult about becoming a young woman or a young man in your family? In your school? In your community? How do you feel about growing up or becoming an adult? In what ways are your life and responsibilities different from the lives and responsibilities of your parents?

Suggested questions for the caregiver of the child or adolescent: *Can you tell me about the child's particular place in the family (e.g., oldest boy, only girl)? Who chose the child's name? Does it have special meaning? Who else is called this? At which ages do you typically expect a child to wean? To walk? To speak? To complete toilet training? What activities do you expect a child of his age to be able to do independently? How do you discipline him? At what age should a child participate in chores? Play alone? Participate in religious observances? Stay home alone? How should a child of his age express respect? What kind of eye contact and physical contact should a child of his age have with adults? How should a child of his age behave around girls? How should he dress around them? What languages are spoken at home? At school? In what ways are religion, spirituality, and community important in family life? How would you expect this child to participate in these activities?*

Early Development and Home Background

If the CFI helps a practitioner understand the cultural background of a young person and their caregivers, the Early Development and Home Background (EDHB) form helps a practitioner assess the risks of adverse childhood experiences (Figures 11–3 and 11–4). Adverse childhood experiences increase the risk of a person experiencing delays in language acquisition (Vernon-Feagans et al. 2012), having fragmentation of identity (Scott et al. 2014), underperforming in educational settings (Romano et al. 2015), and developing substance use disorders (Buu et al. 2009) and mental illnesses (Dvir et al. 2014).

Adverse childhood experiences are common and are associated with profound health outcomes. Approximately 12.5%

Child's Name: _____ **Age:** _____ **Sex:** ☐ Male ☐ Female **Date:** _____

Instructions to Parent or Guardian: Questions P1–P19 ask about the early development and early and current home experiences of your child. Some questions require that you think as far back as to the birth of your child. Your response to these questions will help your child's clinician better understand and care for your child. Answer each question to the best of your knowledge or memory.

What is your relationship with the child receiving care? _____

Please choose one response (✓ or x) for each question.

Early Development	No	Yes	Can't Remember	Don't Know
P1. Was he/she born before he/she was due (premature)?	☐	☐	☐	☐
P2. Were the doctors worried about his/her medical condition immediately after he/she was born?	☐	☐	☐	☐
P3. Did he/she have to spend any time in a neonatal intensive care unit (NICU)?	☐	☐	☐	☐
P4. Could he/she walk on his/her own by the age of 18 months?	☐	☐	☐	☐
P5. Has he/she ever had a seizure?	☐	☐	☐	☐
P6. Did he/she ever lose consciousness for more than a few minutes after an accident?	☐	☐	☐	☐

FIGURE 11–3. Early Development and Home Background (EDHB) form—Parent/Guardian.

Early Communication	No	Yes	Can't Remember	Don't Know
P7. By the time he/she was age 2, could he/she put several words together when speaking?	☐	☐	☐	☐
P8. Could people who didn't know him/her understand his/her speech by the time he/she reached age 4?	☐	☐	☐	☐
P9. Have you ever been concerned about his/her hearing or eyesight?	☐	☐	☐	☐
P10. By the time he/she was age 4, was he/she interested in playing with or being with other children?	☐	☐	☐	☐

FIGURE 11–3. Early Development and Home Background (EDHB) form—Parent/Guardian. *(continued)*

Home Environment	No	Yes	Can't Remember	Don't Know
P11. Was there ever a time when he/she could not live at home and someone else had to look after him/her?	☐	☐		☐
P12. Has he/she ever been admitted to the hospital for a serious illness?	☐	☐	☐	☐
P13. Does anyone at home suffer from a serious health problem?	☐	☐		☐
P14. Does anyone at home have a problem with depression?	☐	☐		☐
P15. Does anyone at home regularly see a counselor, therapist, or other mental health professional?	☐	☐		☐
P16. Does anyone at home have a problem with alcohol, drugs, or other substances?	☐	☐		☐
P17. Would you say that the atmosphere at home is usually pretty calm?	☐	☐		☐
	Less Than Once a Month	Between Once a Week and Once a Month	More Than Once a Week	Most Days
P18. How often are there fights or arguments between people at home?	☐	☐	☐	☐
P19. How often does your child get criticized to his/her face by other family members when he/she is at home?	☐	☐	☐	☐

FIGURE 11–3. Early Development and Home Background (EDHB) form—Parent/Guardian. *(continued)*

(This form is to be completed if this is your FIRST encounter with the child receiving care)

Child's Name: _____ Age: _____ Sex: ☐ Male ☐ Female Date: _____

GENERAL INSTRUCTIONS: The Early Development and Home Background (EDHB) form is used for the assessment of the early development and past and current home background experiences of the child receiving care. The form consists of two versions: 1) 19 P-items, to be completed by the child's parent or guardian, and 2) 8 C-items (herein), to be completed by the clinician. First, the P-items should be completed by the child's parent or guardian. This can be done independently, prior to meeting with the clinician, or be administered to the parent or guardian by the clinician during the clinical interview with the parent's or guardian's response to each question recorded verbatim. Next, the clinician is asked to complete the C-items after a thorough review of the parent's or guardian's responses, ask follow-up questions if necessary, and review any additional clinical information that is available.

Please review the responses provided by the child's parent or guardian for items P1–P10 and then, based on all the information available (i.e., parent/guardian's responses, other information available, and information obtained from the clinical interview), complete questions C1–C4 below			
Early CNS Problems			
C1.	Is there a history suggestive of early neurological damage?	☐ No	☐ Yes	☐ *Unsure*
If yes, specify:			
C2.	Does history suggest delayed language development?	☐ No	☐ Yes	☐ *Unsure*
C3.	Does history suggest possible persistent problems with vision or hearing?	☐ No	☐ Yes	☐ *Unsure*
C4.	Does history suggest early difficulties in social relationships?	☐ No	☐ Yes	☐ *Unsure*
If yes to any, elaborate:			

FIGURE 11–4. Early Development and Home Background form—Clinician.

Please review the responses provided by the child's parent or guardian for items P11-P16 and then, based on all the information available (i.e., parent/guardian's responses, other information available, and information obtained from the clinical interview), complete questions C5a-d below.

Early Disturbances of Home Environment: Early Abuse or Neglect

C5.	Does history suggest early....			
a.	physical abuse?	☐ No	☐ Yes	☐ *Unsure*
b.	sexual abuse?	☐ No	☐ Yes	☐ *Unsure*
c.	neglect?	☐ No	☐ Yes	☐ *Unsure*
d.	damaging nurturance (e.g. frequent change of caregiver)?	☐ No	☐ Yes	☐ *Unsure*

If yes to any, elaborate:

FIGURE 11–4. Early Development and Home Background form—Clinician. *(continued)*

Please review the response provided by the child's parent or guardian for items P13-P19 and then, based on all the information available (i.e., parent/guardian's responses, other information available, and information obtained from the clinical interview), complete questions C6-C8 below.

Home Environment

C6.	Levels of expressed emotion (arguments, expressions of dislike among family members, or criticism of child's behavior, feelings, or individual characteristics) at home are probably ...	☐ Normal	☐ Somewhat High	☐ High	☐ Very High / ☐ *Unsure*
C7.	Is parent/caregiver currently depressed?	☐ No	☐ Somewhat but Mild	☐ Significant	☐ Severe / ☐ *Unsure*

IF ANY ANSWER OTHER THAN "NO" TO QUESTION 7:

C8.	If depressed, is parent/caregiver receiving treatment?	☐ No	☐ Yes	☐ *Unsure*

FIGURE 11–4. Early Development and Home Background form—Clinician. (*continued*)

of the U.S. general public reports experiencing 4 or more of the following 10 adverse childhood experiences: emotional, physical, or sexual abuse; emotional neglect; physical neglect; physically aggressive mother; household substance abuse; household mental illness; parental separation or divorce; and incarceration of a household member. Researchers have linked exposure to such adversities to long-term changes in self-care and health behaviors. Persons exposed to 4 or more different types of adverse childhood experiences are more than twice as likely as those without such experiences to have a stroke, twice as likely to have ischemic heart disease, 4 times as likely to use illicit substances, 7 times as likely to develop alcoholism, and 12 times as likely to attempt suicide. Improving a child's early household experiences therefore is believed to improve their long-term physical health (Hughes et al. 2017).

Practitioners often neglect to assess for a history of adverse childhood experiences. After all, keeping up with the demands of the current encounter with a child or an adolescent is challenging enough without also keeping up with events from the past. We encourage you to develop strategies for assessing adverse experiences, both because of the possibility that adverse experiences may be ongoing and because of the certainty that the sequelae of any adverse experiences are still being worked out by the patient. Either way, you will be able to intervene only if you first identify the adverse experiences. Using the EDHB is one way to do so.

The EDHB is a pair of single-page questionnaires that a practitioner administers sequentially. A caregiver should complete the 19-question version, which assesses development, communication, and the home environment, before (or while) the practitioner meets with the patient. The 8-question version, which assesses early central nervous system problems, early disturbances in a child's life, and the current home environment, should be completed in an interview of the caregiver. The EDHB can be reproduced, without additional permission, for a practitioner's clinical use.

Personality Inventory for DSM-5-TR— Brief Form—Child Age 11–17

During the decade of work preceding the publication of DSM-5, most observers anticipated that the personality disorders would be substantially revised. After all, the categorical model of personality disorders has several known problems: many persons with mental illness have symptoms that meet the criteria for several different personality disorders, practitioners often use personality diagnoses pejoratively, the clustering of personality disorders has little biological basis, and the categorical model does not allow for the identification of character traits that affect function without constituting a full disorder.

To address these concerns, the authors of DSM-5 created a dimensional model of personality disorders. Unlike a categorical model, in which a clinician diagnoses a disorder on the basis of the presence of symptoms that negatively affect functioning, in the dimensional model, a clinician first assesses whether a person has significant deficits in self-functioning and interpersonal functioning before identifying the character traits associated with the functional deficits.

The organizing principle behind the dimensional model of personality disorders is called the *five factors*. In the literature, *five-factor model* usually refers to the adaptive personality traits of neuroticism, extroversion, agreeableness, conscientiousness, and openness to experience (Digman 1990). Because the DSM-5 Work Group built these diagnostic criteria from a deficit-based rather than a strengths-based model, they organized personality disorders around five companion maladaptive traits: negative affect, detachment, antagonism, disinhibition, and psychoticism. The authors found compelling evidence for these five maladaptive traits as stable and predictive of problems in self-functioning and interpersonal functioning. In addition, they identified *facets* for each of these five maladaptive traits. In total, they enumerated 25 facets organized into five domains for each of the maladaptive traits listed earlier in this section. The model was accompanied by a Level of Personality Functioning Scale and Personality Trait Rating Form, with which a clinician could rate the severity of functional impairment and specify a person's maladaptive traits.

If that sounds complicated to you, you are not alone. In the initial version of DSM-5, the dimensional model of personality disorders was tabled in favor of the customary categorical models, with 10 personality disorders organized into Clusters A, B, and C. However, the dimensional model was included in Section III, "Emerging Measures and Models," along with other tools. Many observers believe that a simplified version of the dimensional model for personality disorders will ultimately displace the categorical model.

In the meantime, the authors of DSM-5-TR have encouraged clinicians to use various tools generated during the creation of the dimensional model for personality disorders. It is intriguing that one of those models is of particular interest to clinicians who care for children and adolescents. Unlike the categorical model, which is designed only for adults, whose personalities have been traditionally viewed as more solidified (unlike the actively developing personalities of youth), the dimensional model allows a clinician to assess for self-functioning and interpersonal functioning and specific maladaptive traits in a young person between ages 11 and 17.

The Personality Inventory for DSM-5-TR is available in versions for both adults and children. The full version for children includes 220 questions to be self-completed by the child or adolescent being evaluated. This version is best used in mental health specialty practices and is available online at www.psychiatry.org/psychiatrists/practice/dsm/educational-resources/assessment-measures.

There is also a brief self-administered version, with only 25 questions, which could be used in general settings by interested clinicians. This version can be used to assess a young person's personality traits over time. The Personality Inventory for DSM-5-TR—Brief Form (Figure 11–5) assesses the five personality trait domains described earlier—negative affect, detachment, antagonism, disinhibition, and psychoticism—along with their associated facets.

To score the Personality Inventory for DSM-5-TR—Brief Form, sum the patient's responses. Possible scores range from 0 to 75, with higher scores indicating greater overall personality dysfunction. Further scoring information is available online.

Name: _____ Age: _____ Sex: ☐ Male ☐ Female Date: _____

Instructions: This is a list of things different people might say about themselves. We are interested in how you would describe yourself. There are no right or wrong answers. So you can describe yourself as honestly as possible, we will keep your responses confidential. We'd like you to take your time and read each statement carefully, selecting the response that best describes you.

		Very False or Often False	Sometimes or Somewhat False	Sometimes or Somewhat True	Very True or Often True	Clinician Use Item score
1	People would describe me as reckless.	0	1	2	3	
2	I feel like I act totally on impulse.	0	1	2	3	
3	Even though I know better, I can't stop making rash decisions.	0	1	2	3	
4	I often feel like nothing I do really matters.	0	1	2	3	
5	Others see me as irresponsible.	0	1	2	3	
6	I'm not good at planning ahead.	0	1	2	3	
7	My thoughts often don't make sense to others.	0	1	2	3	
8	I worry about almost everything.	0	1	2	3	
9	I get emotional easily, often for very little reason.	0	1	2	3	
10	I fear being alone in life more than anything else.	0	1	2	3	

FIGURE 11–5. The Personality Inventory for DSM-5-TR—Brief Form (PID-5-BF)—Child Age 11–17.

		Very False or Often False	Sometimes or Somewhat False	Sometimes or Somewhat True	Very True or Often True	Item score
11	I get stuck on one way of doing things, even when it's clear it won't work.	0	1	2	3	
12	I have seen things that weren't really there.	0	1	2	3	
13	I steer clear of romantic relationships.	0	1	2	3	
14	I'm not interested in making friends.	0	1	2	3	
15	I get irritated easily by all sorts of things.	0	1	2	3	
16	I don't like to get too close to people.	0	1	2	3	
17	It's no big deal if I hurt other peoples' feelings.	0	1	2	3	
18	I rarely get enthusiastic about anything.	0	1	2	3	
19	I crave attention.	0	1	2	3	
20	I often have to deal with people who are less important than me.	0	1	2	3	

FIGURE 11–5. The Personality Inventory for DSM-5-TR—Brief Form (PID-5-BF)—Child Age 11–17. (*continued*)

		Very False or Often False	Sometimes or Somewhat False	Sometimes or Somewhat True	Very True or Often True	Item score
21	I often have thoughts that make sense to me but that other people say are strange.	0	1	2	3	
22	I use people to get what I want.	0	1	2	3	
23	I often "zone out" and then suddenly come to and realize that a lot of time has passed.	0	1	2	3	
24	Things around me often feel unreal, or more real than usual.	0	1	2	3	
25	It is easy for me to take advantage of others.	0	1	2	3	
					Total/Partial Raw Score:	
					Prorated Total Score: (if 1–6 items left unanswered)	
					Average Total Score:	

FIGURE 11–5. The Personality Inventory for DSM-5-TR—Brief Form (PID-5-BF)—Child Age 11–17. *(continued)*

Chapter 12

Using Rating Scales and Alternative Diagnostic Systems While Assessing a Young Person

There are many ways you can describe and measure mental distress. When you use DSM-5-TR (American Psychiatric Association 2022), you identify a group of co-occurring signs and symptoms that impair a patient's psychosocial functioning. These functionally impairing signs and symptoms follow each other in predictable ways, and we call these collections *mental disorders*. DSM-5-TR mental disorders are categories rather than discrete biological phenomena. Patients with the same diagnosis often have very different experiences, symptoms, and functional impairments. One adolescent with major depressive disorder may need a course of cognitive-behavioral therapy, whereas another may need hospitalization. To account for these differences, we measure a young person's areas of mental distress with rating scales. Sometimes, we use alternative diagnostic systems to describe the distress differently.

Rating Scales

Because we cannot yet reliably diagnose and monitor mental illness through means such as physical diagnosis, functional imaging, genetic testing, or blood serum tests, rating scales are important aids to clinical care. Individual item responses on a rating scale can be used to guide a clinical conversation: *"You indicated that you sometimes have thoughts that you would be better off dead. Can you tell me more about that?"* Numerical scores on rating scales can be used to identify symptoms, guide diagnostic assessments, establish the severity of a disorder, and track the progress of a young person's care. Collecting rating scale results over time also enables measurement-based care, in which a patient's treatment plan is adjusted until a measurable symptom target is reached.

We follow a few principles when considering how to use rating scales:

- Select scales that are research validated for age, condition, and (ideally) culture and identity.
- Use broad-based screening scales to detect the likelihood of any disorder being present.
- Use a more specific rating scale to investigate a particular problem.
- Select brief rating scales to enhance patient cooperation and ease of implementation.
- Reserve longer rating scales for specialty settings.
- Remember that rating scales cannot make diagnoses—they aid, but cannot replace, clinician assessments.
- Remember that rating scale results depend on the reliability of the reporter and their interpretation.

Many scales are copyrighted by their authors and thus are not freely available. Table 12–1 contains a list of freely available rating scales in common use that have been re-search validated for use with young people. In this context, validity means that each scale has a research-supported scoring system that balances the need for good sensitivity (the test detects most patients who have a disorder) with good specificity (the test is positive only when a disorder is present).

DSM-5-TR provides severity rating scales for many disorders. Most of these scales are specific to a particular disorder, and some include a narrative description to indicate that the disorder is mild, moderate, or severe. For some diagnoses, such as alcohol use disorder, severity depends on the number of criteria endorsed by a patient. For others, such as body dysmorphic disorder, severity depends on the patient's degree of insight. In other instances, severity is measured by the degree to which a patient requires support, as in autism spectrum disorder. When appropriate, the severity ratings refer to specific measurements external to your mental status examination. For example, one potential aspect of assessing the severity of intellectual disability entails assessing a patient's IQ, and one aspect of assessing the severity of anorexia nervosa entails assessing BMI.

TABLE 12–1. Selected brief rating scales that are validated and free to use with children and adolescents

Category	Scale	Number of items	Validated ages for use (years)
Overall psychosocial difficulties	Pediatric Symptom Checklist (PSC, PSC-17)	Parent: 35 or 17 Youth: 35	4–17 (parent version) 11–17 (youth version)
	Strengths and Difficulties Questionnaire (SDQ)	Parent: 25	4–16
Global functioning	Columbia Impairment Scale	Parent: 13 Youth: 13	9–17
	Brief Impairment Scale	Parent: 21	4–17
Behavior and emotional development	Early Childhood Screening Assessment (ECSA)	Parent: 40	1.5–5
Anxiety	Screen for Child Anxiety Related Disorders (SCARED)	Parent and youth: 41	9–17
	Spence Children's Anxiety Scale (SCAS)	Parent: 39 Youth: 45	6–17

TABLE 12–1. Selected brief rating scales that are validated and free to use with children and adolescents *(continued)*

Category	Scale	Number of items	Validated ages for use (years)
	Spence Preschool Anxiety Scale	Parent: 39	3–5
Depression	Short Mood and Feelings Questionnaire (SMFQ)	Parent: 13 Youth: 13	8–17
	Patient Health Questionnaire–9 (PHQ-9)	Youth: 9	13–17
	Center for Epidemiological Studies Depression Scale for Children (CES-DC)	Youth: 20	13–17
ADHD	Vanderbilt ADHD Diagnostic Parent Rating Scale/Vanderbilt ADHD Diagnostic Teacher Rating Scale	Parent: 55 Teacher: 43	6–12
	SNAP-IV-C Rating Scale	Parent/teacher: 90	6–17
	ADHD Rating Scale–IV	Parent/teacher: 18	6–17
Schizophrenia	10-Item Pediatric Positive and Negative Symptoms Scale	Youth: 10	13–17

TABLE 12–1. Selected brief rating scales that are validated and free to use with children and adolescents *(continued)*

Category	Scale	Number of items	Validated ages for use (years)
PTSD	Children's Revised Impact of Events Scale–8 (CRIES-8)	Youth: 8	8–17
Substance use	CRAFFT (Car, Relax, Alone, Forget, Friends, Trouble)	Youth: 6	13–17
Autism spectrum disorder	Modified Checklist for Autism in Toddlers (M-CHAT)	Parent: 23	16–30 months
	Childhood Autism Spectrum Test (CAST)	Parent: 39	4–11
	Autism-Spectrum Quotient (AQ)	Parent: 50	12–15
Maternal depression	Edinburgh Postnatal Depression Scale (EPDS)	Parent: 10	Peripartum women

The authors of DSM-5-TR have posted several disorder-specific severity measures (Table 12–2) at www.psychiatry.org/psychiatrists/practice/dsm/educational-resources/assessment-measures. These measures can be used (and reproduced) for clinical and research evaluation without further permission. A practitioner who frequently cares for children and adolescents with these specific conditions should consider using them in their practice.

Alternative Diagnostic Systems

Although DSM-5-TR provides a common vocabulary for characterizing mental distress, various communities use alternative vocabularies when describing the experiences of a person experiencing mental distress or illness (Clark et al. 2017).

Culture-Specific Diagnostic Systems

The experience of mental illness and distress is always mediated through culture, which structures the human experience of health, illness, and receiving care. DSM-5-TR renews attention to the roles culture plays in mental disorders, building on the development of the Cultural Formulation Interview, which is included in Chapter 11, "Using DSM-5-TR Assessment Measures to Aid Diagnosis," and can be explored extensively elsewhere (Lewis-Fernández et al. 2016). Outside of DSM-5-TR, culture-specific psychiatric diagnostic systems are used in China (Chen 2002), Cuba (Otero-Ojeda 2002), Japan (Nakane and Nakane 2002), and Latin America (Berganza and Mezzich 2004) and can be seen in specific faith traditions such as Islam (Keshavarzi et al. 2020). There is also a French diagnostic system specifically designed for use with children and adolescents (Mises et al. 2002).

International Classification of Diseases

Across cultures, the World Health Organization maintains its own descriptive diagnostic system, the International Statistical Classification of Diseases and Related Health Problems, commonly called the International Classification of Diseases (ICD). The 11th revision (ICD-11) includes mental disorders within a catalog of all medical diseases. Although most clinicians outside the United States use ICD-11 to diagnose men-

TABLE 12–2. DSM-5-TR disorder-specific severity measures for children and adolescents ages 11–17 years

Rater	Scale	Number of items	Source measure
Self	Severity Measure for Depression	9	Adapted from Patient Health Questionnaire–9 (PHQ-9) modified for adolescents (PHQ-A)
Self	Severity Measure for Separation Anxiety Disorder	10	Each anxiety severity scale contains the same 10 items, with a few adaptations to phrasing to match the DSM-5 criteria for each disorder
Self	Severity Measure for Specific Phobia	10	
Self	Severity Measure for Social Anxiety Disorder (Social Phobia)	10	
Self	Severity Measure for Panic Disorder	10	
Self	Severity Measure for Agoraphobia	10	
Self	Severity Measure for Generalized Anxiety Disorder	10	

TABLE 12–2. DSM-5-TR disorder-specific severity measures for children and adolescents ages 11–17 years *(continued)*

Rater	Scale	Number of items	Source measure
Self	Severity of Posttraumatic Stress Symptoms	9	National Stressful Events Survey PTSD Short Scale (NSESS)
Self	Severity of Acute Stress Symptoms	7	National Stressful Events Survey Acute Stress Disorder Short Scale (NSESS)
Self	Severity of Dissociative Symptoms	8	Brief Dissociative Experiences Scale (DES-B)
Practitioner	Clinician-Rated Severity of Autism Spectrum and Social Communication Disorders	2	Uses DSM-5 autism severity descriptions
Practitioner	Clinician-Rated Dimensions of Psychosis Symptom Severity	8	Not adapted: appears in Section III of DSM-5
Practitioner	Clinician-Rated Severity of Somatic Symptom Disorder	3	Derived from DSM-5 disorder diagnostic criteria
Practitioner	Clinician-Rated Severity of Oppositional Defiant Disorder	1	Uses DSM-5 oppositional defiant disorder severity description

TABLE 12–2. DSM-5-TR disorder-specific severity measures for children and adolescents ages 11–17 years (*continued*)

Rater	Scale	Number of items	Source measure
Practitioner	Clinician-Rated Severity of Conduct Disorder	1	Uses DSM-5 conduct disorder severity description
Practitioner	Clinician-Rated Severity of Nonsuicidal Self-Injury	1	Derived from DSM-5 diagnostic threshold for proposed nonsuicidal self-injury disorder

tal disorders, ICD-11 was primarily designed to help epidemiologists track the incidence and prevalence of disease for public health interventions, so it provides less information for each diagnosis than does DSM-5-TR. Despite their different designs, DSM-5-TR and ICD-11 assign essentially the same codes to psychiatric diagnoses, and these shared codes are widely used by insurers and regulators. The sixth chapter of ICD-11, "Mental, Behavioural or Neurodevelopmental Disorders," includes most of the diagnoses relevant for a diagnostic interview. However, sleep-wake disorders, sexual dysfunctions, and gender incongruence are coded in other chapters of ICD-11. Some clinicians may prefer ICD-11 because it is freely available online, is commonly used in electronic health records, provides diagnostic guidelines rather than the comparatively stricter criteria sets of DSM-5-TR, maintains a distinction between substance abuse and dependence, and has moved gender incongruence out of its list of mental disorders and into its "Conditions Related to Sexual Health" chapter. Information about ICD-11 can be found at https://icd.who.int/browse11/l-m/en.

Hierarchical Taxonomy of Psychopathology

The Hierarchical Taxonomy of Psychopathology (HiTOP) uses dimensions to cut across DSM-5-TR diagnostic categories. The mental health clinicians and researchers who crafted the HiTOP came from a broad range of theoretical perspectives. Their goal was to create a nosology acknowledging that mental health exists along a spectrum between normal and pathological. So instead of a categorical model that declares that a person does or does not have, say, ADHD, the HiTOP recognizes that clinical impairments in attention are related to the fluctuations in attention and activity that everyone experiences. The HiTOP also allows clinicians to diagnose a person across existing diagnostic categories. For example, the HiTOP recognizes the evidence for similarities between ADHD and conduct disorder. Finally, the taxonomy allows for a clinician to see the relationship between a symptom and its constituent components, such as maladaptive traits and externalizing behavior. So instead of just diagnosing a person with ADHD, a clinician can identify a disinhibited person engaged in antisocial behavior with associated signs, symptoms, and maladaptive behaviors. The HiTOP model is designed to be evidence based, reliable, and valid, but it is not yet commonly used (Kotov et al. 2017). To get a sense of how it works, a clinician could trial the dimensional model of personality disorders described in Section III of DSM-5-TR, which it resembles.

Power Threat Meaning Framework

The HiTOP, like DSM-5-TR and ICD-11, characterizes the specific mental illness of a particular person. However, no person experiences mental illness or mental health alone. A group of British psychologists, aided by persons with mental illness, developed the Power Threat Meaning Framework (PTM) to consider how the person, their family, and their social groups affect the person's mental health. The authors of the PTM observed that in contemporary life we medicalize aspects of human distress. We diagnose a person as "depressed" instead of, say, naming the domestic violence that precipitated a depressive episode. The PTM is not a full diagnostic system, but it is a powerful way to engage a person who is experiencing mental distress. A clinician can incorporate some of the PTM's insights into a diagnostic interview by including four questions (Johnstone et al. 2018, p. 9):

1. What has happened to you? (How is power operating in your life?)
2. How did it affect you? (What kind of threats does this pose?)
3. What sense did you make of it? (What is the meaning of these situations and experiences to you?)
4. What did you have to do to survive? (What kinds of threat responses are you using?)

The PTM also offers questions to help a patient think about their resources and develop their experiences into a narrative. For example, the following two questions could be profitably included by a clinician in a diagnostic interview (Johnstone et al. 2018, p. 246):

1. What are your strengths? (What access to power resources do you have?)
2. What is your story? (How does all this fit together?)

As these questions suggest, the PTM provides a thoughtful way to engage the agency of a person experiencing mental distress and to contextualize their experience within their relationships and their narrative understanding of their life.

Research Domain Criteria

In its own attempts to pursue the cause of mental illness, the National Institute of Mental Health is producing the Research Domain Criteria (RDoC; Insel et al. 2010). At present, RDoC serves as an experimental framework for researching the biological origin of psychiatric illness, but its goal differs from that of DSM-5 (American Psychiatric Association 2013; see Clark et al. 2017). The goal of this project is to map behavioral patterns onto etiological cells, genes, molecules, and neural circuits for which new research and new treatments could be developed rather than relying on traditional clinical diagnosis. In this way, a specific pattern might be found through RDoC to have a relatively unified underlying biological cause (Kozak and Cuthbert 2016). DSM-5-TR takes an important step in the direction of RDoC because it includes dimensions—which are analogous to what RDoC calls behavioral "domains"—such as impulsivity and negative emotionality, cut across contemporary diagnostic categories, and renews consideration of the etiology of mental distress (Insel and Quirion 2005). The development of RDoC can be followed online (www.nimh.nih.gov/research/research-funded-by-nimh/rdoc).

Diagnostic Systems for Infants and Toddlers

Several diagnostic systems exist for assessing psychopathology in very young children (Egger and Emde 2011). The most widely used, the *Diagnostic Classification of Mental Health and Developmental Disorders of Infancy and Early Childhood*, has evolved into the current version (DC:0–5), which covers up to age 5 (Zero to Three 2016). It uses a multiaxis system as in DSM-IV (American Psychiatric Association 1994) but is shaped around describing infant relationships and problematic behavior patterns. The Research Diagnostic Criteria—Preschool Age (RDC-PA) was designed for the evaluation of children ages 0–5 years participating in behavioral health research (Task Force on Research Diagnostic Criteria: Infancy Preschool 2003).

ICD-11 Z Codes

DSM-5 recommends the use of ICD-11 Z codes as a way to account for the psychosocial factors that are currently affecting a young person's mental health and treatment. ICD-10 Z codes are discussed further in Chapter 14, "Crafting Pediatric Mental Health Treatment Plans," but we include an abbreviated list of ICD-11 Z codes here in Table 12–3.

TABLE 12–3. ICD-11 codes commonly used in child and adolescent mental health

ICD-11 code	Description
Z00.4	General psychiatric examination, not elsewhere classified
	Exclusion: examination requested for medicolegal reasons (Z04.6)
Z04.6	General psychiatric examination, requested by authority
Z30.0	General counseling and advice on contraception
Z33	Pregnant state, incidental
Z50.2	Alcohol rehabilitation
Z50.3	Drug rehabilitation
Z50.4	Psychotherapy, not elsewhere classified
Z51.5	Palliative care
Z55.0	Illiteracy and low-level literacy
Z55.3	Underachievement in school
Z55.4	Educational maladjustment and discord with teachers and classmates
Z55.9	Other problems related to education and literacy
Z59.0	Homelessness
Z59.1	Inadequate housing
Z59.2	Discord with neighbor, lodger, or landlord
Z59.3	Problem related to living in a residential institution
Z59.4	Lack of adequate food or safe drinking water
Z59.5	Extreme poverty
Z59.6	Low income
Z59.7	Insufficient social or health insurance or welfare support
Z79.9	Unspecified housing or economic problem

TABLE 12–3. ICD-11 codes commonly used in child and adolescent mental health *(continued)*

ICD-11 code	Description
Z60.0	Phase of life problem
Z60.3	Acculturation difficulty
Z60.4	Social exclusion or rejection
Z60.5	Target of (perceived) adverse discrimination or persecution
Z60.9	Other problem related to social environment
Z61.0	Loss of love relationship in childhood
Z61.1	Removal from home in childhood
Z61.2	Altered pattern of family relationships in childhood
Z61.3	Events resulting in loss of self-esteem in childhood
Z61.4	Problems related to alleged sexual abuse of child by person within primary support group
Z61.5	Problems related to alleged sexual abuse of child by person outside primary support group
Z61.6	Problems related to alleged physical abuse of child
Z61.7	Personal frightening experience in childhood
Z62.0	Inadequate parental supervision and control
Z62.1	Parental overprotection
Z62.2	Institutional upbringing
Z62.4	Emotional neglect of child
Z62.820	Parent-child relational problem
Z62.891	Sibling relational problem
Z62.29	Upbringing away from parents
Z62.810	Personal history (past history) of physical abuse in childhood

TABLE 12–3. ICD-11 codes commonly used in child and adolescent mental health *(continued)*

ICD-11 code	Description
Z62.810	Personal history (past history) of sexual abuse in childhood
Z62.811	Personal history (past history) of psychological abuse in childhood
Z62.812	Personal history (past history) of neglect in childhood
Z62.898	Child affected by parental relationship distress
Z63.1	Problems in relationship with parents and in-laws
Z63.2	Inadequate family support
Z63.4	Uncomplicated bereavement
Z63.5	Disruption of family by separation or divorce
Z63.6	Dependent relative needing care at home
Z63.8	High expressed emotion level within family
Z64.0	Problems related to unwanted pregnancy
Z64.1	Problems related to multiparity
Z64.2	Seeking and accepting physical, nutritional and chemical interventions known to be hazardous and harmful Exclusion: substance dependence
Z64.3	Seeking and accepting behavioral and psychological interventions known to be hazardous and harmful
Z64.4	Discord with social service provider, including probation officer, case manager, or social services worker
Z65.0	Conviction in civil or criminal proceedings without imprisonment
Z65.1	Imprisonment or other incarceration
Z65.2	Problems related to release from prison

TABLE 12–3. ICD-11 codes commonly used in child and adolescent mental health *(continued)*

ICD-11 code	Description
Z65.3	Problems related to other legal circumstances
Z65.4	Victim of crime or terrorism
Z65.5	Exposure to disaster, war, or other hostilities
Z65.8	Other problem related to psychosocial circumstances
Z65.8	Religious or spiritual problem
Z65.9	Unspecified problem related to unspecified psychosocial circumstances
Z69.010	Encounter for mental health services for victim of child abuse or neglect by parent
Z69.020	Encounter for mental health services for victim of nonparental child abuse or neglect
Z70.3	Counseling related to combined concerns regarding sexual attitude, behavior and orientation
Z71.1	Person with feared complaint in whom no diagnosis is made
Z71.4	Alcohol abuse counseling and surveillance
	Exclusion: alcohol rehabilitation procedures
Z71.5	Drug abuse counseling and surveillance
	Exclusion: drug rehabilitation procedures
Z71.6	Tobacco abuse counseling
	Exclusion: tobacco rehabilitation procedures
Z72.0	Tobacco use disorder, mild
Z72.1	Alcohol use
	Exclusion: alcohol dependence
Z72.2	Drug use

ICD-11 code	Description
	Exclusion: abuse of non-dependence-producing substances, drug dependence
Z72.3	Lack of physical exercise
Z72.4	Inappropriate diet and eating habits
	Exclusion: eating disorder or lack of food
Z72.5	High-risk sexual behavior
Z72.810	Child or adolescent antisocial behavior
Z73.6	Limitation of activities due to disability
	Exclusion: care-provider dependency
Z74.0	Reduced mobility
Z74.1	Need for assistance with personal care
Z74.3	Need for continuous supervision
Z75.1	Person awaiting admission to adequate facility elsewhere
Z75.3	Unavailability or inaccessibility of health care facilities
Z75.4	Unavailability or inaccessibility of other helping agencies
Z76.5	Malingering
Z91.1	Personal history of noncompliance with medical treatment and regimen
Z91.199	Nonadherence to medical treatment
Z91.2	Personal history of poor personal hygiene
Z91.3	Personal history of unhealthy sleep-wake schedule
Z91.49	Other personal history of psychological trauma
Z91.5	Personal history of self-harm
Z91.6	Personal history of other physical trauma

TABLE 12–3. ICD-11 codes commonly used in child and adolescent mental health *(continued)*

ICD-11 code	Description
Z91.83	Wandering associated with a mental disorder
	Child neglect, confirmed
T74.02XA	Initial encounter
T74.02XD	Subsequent encounter
	Child neglect, suspected
T76.02XA	Initial encounter
T76.02XD	Subsequent encounter
	Child psychological abuse, confirmed
T74.32XA	Initial encounter
T74.32XD	Subsequent encounter
	Child psychological abuse, suspected
T76.32XA	Initial encounter
T76.32XD	Subsequent encounter
	Child sexual abuse, confirmed
T74.22XA	Initial encounter
T74.22XD	Subsequent encounter
	Child sexual abuse, suspected
T76.22XA	Initial encounter
T76.22XD	Subsequent encounter

Chapter 13

Recognizing Developmental Red Flags

Observations of child maturation by developmental theorists are foundational for pediatrics, child psychiatry, and child psychology. The work of many different theorists over the years (e.g., Beloglovsky and Daly 2015; McCartney and Philips 2006; Mooney 2013) has resulted in a diverse set of theories about what happens during child development. Although a survey of this literature is beyond the scope of this text, we can discuss specific observable milestones within child development and their recognized patterns of appearance.

Milestones are recognizable skills or abilities with an expected range and order of appearance, such as a child taking their first step around the time of their first birthday. Identifying any significant variations from expected patterns, such as a child only taking their first step near their second birthday, is a key task for any practitioner. Knowing when a significant variation in development has occurred improves diagnostic accuracy because DSM-5-TR (American Psychiatric Association 2022) specifically requires consideration of developmental stages. The sooner a significant developmental impairment is identified and addressed, the better the long-term outcomes for your patients.

Identifying milestones is a particularly important skill set for practitioners working with children younger than 5 years, but we all need to be familiar with milestones because nonsevere developmental impairments frequently go unrecognized until children are much older. Five different milestone skill areas should be evaluated: gross and fine motor, visual motor problem-solving, speech and language, social and emotional, and adaptive skills (Gerber et al. 2011).

Gross motor skills are the most obvious to recognize because they involve crawling, walking, running, and throwing. Early motor skills are related to performing basic body control tasks, starting with first maintaining a head position, then moving the trunk, followed by moving the whole body in ever more skillful ways. Besides significant delays in gross motor skills, any physical findings of abnormal reflexes, asymmetric muscle tone, or being too loose or too tight in overall muscle tone are gross motor abnormalities that should be noted.

Visual motor problem-solving describes a child's physical interactions with the world. Infants begin by visually tracking and following people or objects, then reaching for and manipulating objects; later they acquire the ability to draw and to write. These fine motor skills (using one's hands and fingers) rely on visual input and generally progress at a slower pace than gross motor skills. If the development of these milestones is delayed, it may be because of impairments in sensory, cognitive, or motor abilities.

Speech and language skills are essential for social interactions and academic success. To be able to communicate, a person has to be able first to receive input (process what is seen and heard), pragmatically understand the meaning of that input, and then generate an expression of their thoughts (translate thoughts into words, then express them fluently). Delays in expressive language milestones may be more apparent than delays in receptive language, which may be more subtle but when present may worsen an expressive language impairment.

Social-emotional skills are the core elements of psychiatric functioning. Infants are essentially born with three emotions (anger, joy, and fear), and the circumstances to elicit those feelings become increasingly complex as they grow up. Social skill development is interactive and thus reliant on the presence of a responsive caregiver, or it can be negatively impacted by aversive or nonresponsive caregivers. A child's temperamental traits, such as having a high- or low-intensity disposition, influence how they respond to routine activities, which influences how their caregivers respond back in a feedback loop. Developing shared joint attention with another person by approximately age 1 year is a key social milestone. Typical social and emotional development relies on many other skills but is most closely linked with speech and language skills.

Adaptive skills initially involve learning to feed oneself, dress oneself, and use the bathroom. For older children, adaptive skills involve self-direction, self-protection, and the ability to function independently in a school setting. Adaptive skills rely on both motor and cognitive abilities and thus are not a truly independent category of development. When you evaluate for the presence of an intellectual disability, adaptive milestones need to be investigated because the intellectual disability diagnosis should not be made without demonstrable impairments in adaptive functioning. Standardized intelligence testing is not considered the sole basis for diagnosing intellectual disability in the absence of real-world functional impairments.

A child may acquire all their skills in the usual sequence but at a slower rate (a delay), may acquire their skills at differential rates in different areas (a dissociation), or may achieve milestones out of the usual order of acquisition (a deviation). Growth and development tend to follow recognizable patterns, but it is not an exact script. For instance, a perfectly healthy child might never crawl, instead scooting or rolling to move around before taking their first steps. The task of a pediatric health care clinician is to always consider what would constitute normal range development (Table 13–1). Then the clinician can, variously, alert caregivers if a child is not keeping pace with development and thus needs developmental assistance services, or reassure worried caregivers when a child is keeping pace with the normal range of development, or simply better understand how a child engages their environment.

Determining when a child's delayed milestone acquisition indicates the need for further evaluations or an intervention can be challenging when developmental delays are subtle. To guide your decision, Table 13–2 contains a list of specific cognitive, motor, and social-emotional traits at different ages that suggest a need to refer for specialized developmental assessments.

TABLE 13–1. Selected normal-range developmental milestones in the first 5 years of life

Age	Gross motor	Visual motor	Speech and language	Social-emotional	Adaptive skills
2 months	Has good head control; lifts chest up in prone	Tracks with eyes; holds own hands	Is alert to voice; makes vowel-like noises	Shows reciprocal smiling; recognizes parents	Opens mouth at sight of breast or bottle
4 months	Leans on wrists in prone; rolls prone to supine	Has hands usually open; reaches persistently	Orients self to voice; vocalizes in response	Parent's voice stops cry; smiles on own	Briefly holds breast or bottle
6 months	Briefly sits alone; pivots in prone	Rakes item to pick up; transfers hand to hand	Stops briefly for "no"; babbles consonants	Has stranger anxiety; visually identifies parent	Feeds crackers to self; stares at new faces
9 months	Pulls to stand; cruises; comes to sit	Has immature pincer; looks for fallen toy	Imitates sounds; enjoys gesture games	Follows a point; experiences separation anxiety	Bites, chews cookie; looks for fallen item

TABLE 13–1. Selected normal-range developmental milestones in the first 5 years of life *(continued)*

Age	Gross motor	Visual motor	Speech and language	Social-emotional	Adaptive skills
12 months	Stands well; takes independent steps	Has fine pincer grasp; scribbles if shown	Follows one-step request; uses gestures	Points to get object; shows shared interest	Finger-feeds items; takes off a hat
18 months	Runs well; stands for ball throw	Scribbles on own; makes 3-cube tower	Points to self; uses 10–25 words	Can show shame; does pretend play	Gets onto chair; removes garment
2 years	Throws overhand; kicks ball	Makes 4-cube train; imitates circle and line	Uses two-word sentences; understands "me" and "you"	Does parallel play; begins defiance	Opens doorknob; pulls off pants
3 years	Walks up stairs; catches ball	Copies a circle; recognizes a color	Uses three-word sentences; names body parts	Engages in imaginative play; can share on own	Begins independent eating; unbuttons item

TABLE 13–1. Selected normal-range developmental milestones in the first 5 years of life *(continued)*

Age	Gross motor	Visual motor	Speech and language	Social-emotional	Adaptive skills
4 years	Balances on one foot 4 seconds; can broad jump 1 foot	Writes part of name; copies a square	Follows three-step request; tells stories	Group play; has preferred friend	Toilets self alone; uses fork well
5 years	Walks down stairs; jumps backward	Cuts with scissors; uses a paper clip	Responds to "Why?"; likes rhyming words	Apologizes for an error; has group of friends	Dresses and bathes independently

Source.   Adapted from Gerber et al. 2010, 2011; Wilks et al. 2010.

TABLE 13–2. Developmental red flags that should trigger specialized assessments

Age	Cognitive	Motor	Social-emotional
4 months	Lack of visual tracking; no laugh or vocalizations	Lack of seated head control; inability to grasp toy	Does not watch or track people; does not have a smile response
6 months	Failure to turn toward sound or voice	Does not roll or move on the floor	Lack of spontaneous smile
9 months	Lack of babbling consonants	Inability to sit	Cannot reciprocate vocalizations or facial expressions
1 year	Cannot respond to own name; cannot imitate sounds	Cannot hold two objects and hit them together; cannot pull to a stand	Cannot reciprocate hand gestures; will not share joint attention ("Look at….")
1.5 years	Cannot point to a named object; cannot use any words	Unable to walk independently	Lack of any speaking-gesture combinations
2 years	Speech much less than 50% understandable	Cannot walk on steps with assistance; cannot kick a ball	Cannot use a meaningful two-word phrase; lack of empathy (looking sad if a child cries)

TABLE 13–2. Developmental red flags that should trigger specialized assessments (*continued*)

Age	Cognitive	Motor	Social-emotional
3 years	Cannot use a three-word sentence; speech only 50% understandable	Cannot jump; cannot throw object overhand	Never imitates adult activities; cannot do parallel play
4 years	Speech less than 75% understandable; cannot identify self or details in pictures	Cannot balance on one foot for 3 seconds; cannot copy a circle	Lack of imaginative play; cannot hypothesize another's thoughts

Source. Adapted from Gerber et al. 2010, 2011; McLaughlin 2011; Wilks et al. 2010.

Chapter 14

Crafting Pediatric Mental Health Treatment Plans

Clinicians can understand a treatment plan as a regulatory requirement, as one of the many chores of contemporary health care, or as a recipe for changing a patient's life. After all, the goal of any medical intervention is to help a person achieve a therapeutic change they cannot make on their own, so a treatment plan simply names what they need to change, who will help them, and how they will make the change. Any reasonable treatment plan includes a problem list, a list of measurable goals, and a recipe for how to achieve the goals.

The reality, of course, is that although a treatment plan can be a useful recipe, managing one can be a chore. After all, treatment plans are often required by government agencies and third-party payers. Regulators and payers often require the completion of mental health treatment plans in their own proprietary formats. We encourage you to identify treatment plans specific to the requirements of your clinical setting because only those treatment plans fulfill the chore aspect of a treatment plan. In this chapter, we discuss three general principles universal to the useful recipe aspect of treatment plans: problem lists, patient and caregiver goals, and best practices. They are the what, the who, and the how of treatment plans.

Problem Lists

When you evaluate a young person in mental distress, your goal should be to create a therapeutic alliance, but the tangible result of an evaluation is a diagnosis. This diagnosis is the foundation of a treatment plan.

In early versions of DSM, diagnoses were described in a multiaxial, or five-axis, system. Clinicians divided a diagnosis into five components: mental disorders, personality disorders, general medical conditions, psychosocial problems, and global functioning. At its best, the multiaxial system encouraged clinicians to understand a person's distress from several different perspectives: a biological account of mental illness, a psychological account of personality, a mechanistic account of physical illness, a subjective list of psychosocial factors, and a standardized assessment of functioning. At its worst, the multiaxial system reinforced divisions between mind and body; allowed personality disorders to be used as pejorative slurs; included inconsistent accounts of psychosocial functioning; and jumbled together categories, lists, and assessments. It turned out to be a messy recipe.

The authors of DSM-5 (American Psychiatric Association 2013) reorganized the multiaxial system into the problem list widely used throughout medicine: a comprehensive, hierarchical catalog of the problems addressed during a current encounter. To be helpful, the items on the list should be standardized to enable communication. There are many ways to account for mental distress and mental illness. Individual clinicians may focus on dysfunctional neural circuits, adverse childhood experiences, or maladaptive personality traits. When these clinicians wish to speak with each other, they need a standard list. The standard list we favor is DSM-5 because it is the consensus diagnostic system of contemporary psychiatry, our way for mental health clinicians to work together while we await a diagnostic system with greater validity.

One reminder that we are awaiting a diagnostic system with improved validity is that the diagnoses generated by a DSM-5 interview are called *disorders* rather than *diseases* or *illnesses*. Physicians usually think in terms of diseases, which can be described as pathological abnormalities in the structure and function of body organs and systems. Patients usually present with illnesses, their experience of pathological abnormalities or of being sick. From a distance, diseases and illnesses may seem like the same experience viewed from the different perspectives of patient and physician. However, diseases and illnesses are often divergent experiences, not just different perspectives, as anthropologists have repeatedly documented (Estroff and Henderson 2005).

Disorders are a kind of middle path between disease and illness because the term acknowledges the complex interplay of biological, social, cultural, and psychological factors in mental distress. Broadly speaking, a disorder simply indicates a disturbance in physical or psychological functioning.

Using *disorder* to describe mental distress draws attention to how mental distress impairs a person's functioning, suggests the complex interplay of events that results in mental distress, and implicitly acknowledges the limits of our knowledge about the causes of mental distress (Kendler 2012). The field does not yet know enough to be more precise. The ongoing use of *disorder* in our diagnostic systems is an opportunity for humility, a spur to further study, and a way to communicate together.

For DSM-5 to work as a common language, clinicians need to be specific. Imagine a recipe that asks you to add "a serving of fat." Someone following the recipe would be confused. Did the author of the recipe mean a spoonful of bacon drippings, 2 tablespoons of salted butter, or a half cup of coconut oil? Each is possible, but each results in a different dish, and the direction is more of a personal inspiration than a communal instruction that can be followed by others. Similarly, clinicians should recognize that characterizing a young person as having an "unspecified mental disorder" inadequately communicates the precise nature of the patient's illness to other clinicians.

We encourage clinicians to select the most specific diagnosis for which a patient qualifies. If you believe a child is depressed, determine not only whether the depression constitutes a major depressive episode but also whether it is a single or recurrent episode; with or without psychotic features; and mild, moderate, or severe. This level of specificity enables communication with other clinicians and informs their treatment. We recognize the different ways to treat depression in a child if it is a mild first episode rather than a severe recurrent episode with psychotic features, but we barely know how to proceed with a child who has a nonspecific disorder. Identifying a specific disorder improves communication with other clinicians while communicating to your patients (and their caregivers) your diagnostic ability and your understanding of the patient's illness. Diagnosis is, itself, a response to a patient's suffering because giving a specific name to the seemingly unnamable is itself salutary. (It also improves your ability to communicate with regulators and third-party payers, many of whom reimburse better for more specific diagnoses.)

Still, at times, a specific diagnosis is inappropriate. When you are uncertain of the diagnosis or need additional information, a provisional diagnosis is always preferable to a specific but inaccurate diagnosis. Just remember to name what additional information is necessary for you to eventually arrive at a more specific diagnosis. It is discouraging to review medical records in which a young person's diagnosis remains poorly characterized or mislabeled for years.

Even if your diagnoses lack specificity, you can make them comprehensive. They should include all problems that are currently diminishing a young person's ability to function. Thus, the list should include mental disorders, general medical conditions, and psychosocial problems. We use DSM-5 to describe mental disorders, including the adverse effects from psychiatric treatment that are described in Section II of DSM-5. To describe general medical conditions, we include the medical conditions that are currently affecting a young person's function. You do not need to list well-healed injuries. To describe psychosocial problems that influence a young person's health, we favor using the standardized list of ICD-10 Z codes (World Health Organization 1992). Several of the most relevant Z codes are found in Chapter 12 of this book, "Using Rating Scales and Alternative Diagnostic Systems While Assessing a Young Person," but the complete list of Z codes, numbered Z00–Z99, is found in the ICD chapter "Factors Influencing Health Status and Contact With Health Services," which can be found online at https://icd.who.int/browse10/2019/en#/XXI.

Finally, the problems should be ordered hierarchically. Problems that are the focus of your treatment should lead the list. For example, an adolescent may have cystic fibrosis, but if you are treating them for an episode of major depressive disorder following an intentional overdose, then their first two problems are major depressive disorder and a suicide attempt. If you evaluate them again 2 months later and they have recovered from depression and the intentional ingestion, then the depressive episode and suicide attempt will be lower on their problem list. A well-ordered problem list communicates to everyone who reviews your record the current focus of your treatment.

Patient and Caregiver Goals

You develop the goals of your treatment in conversation with your patient and their caregivers. Sometimes clinicians ask about goals toward the end of a clinical conversation. We prefer to ask about goals from the beginning and then throughout the conversation. Asking about goals is another way to establish a therapeutic alliance, the mutual commitment you and a patient make to improve their well-being. You and the patient establish the alliance when the patient identifies treatment goals and you ally yourself with them in pursuit of those goals. By doing this early in your encounter, you invariably increase the amount and reliability of information a patient offers. More profoundly, you help motivate the patient's desire to change. We ask, often very directly, "*What is your treatment goal?*" or with younger children, "*If you had three magic wishes, what would you change about your life?*" Then, as the encounter progresses, we frequently check on additional goals, saying something like, "*I hear that you are concerned; should we address that as a treatment goal?*" or for smaller children, "*Is that the kind of thing you would use a magic wish on?*" By continuing to ask about treatment goals, a practitioner clarifies the focus of treatment and further builds the alliance with a patient.

By the end of a conversation in which you have frequently asked about treatment goals, it is usually straightforward to summarize the most pressing goals. We often do this by saying, "*It sounds like we have identified the most important treatment goals, but I want to be certain. Have we identified the right goals?*" or with a younger child, "*I think I know what you would use your three wishes on, but I want to check with you and be sure.*" These kinds of conversations ensure that your treatment goals reflect the patient's desire, which usually increases their interest in pursuing the goals. When possible and appropriate, phrase the treatment goals in the patient's own words.

Part of the challenge of working with children and adolescents with mental distress is bringing patients and caregivers together in pursuit of common goals. With patients, we prefer to identify goals early in an encounter. With caregivers, we like to understand the relationship between the caregiver and the patient before asking about treatment goals. Different caregivers are invested in patients in different ways. Is the caregiver a biological parent, stepparent, foster parent, grandparent, older sibling, guardian, probation officer, or teacher? These relationships affect the treatment goals a caregiver identifies and their ability to affect those goals. If, say, an adolescent presents for treatment with their probation officer, the treatment goals will likely include legal requirements, which are quite different from the patient's goals. You need to know how and why a caregiver is involved in a young person's life before soliciting the caregiver's treatment goals.

Once the patient, caregiver, and practitioner agree on treatment goals, it helps to consider the settings in which the goals will be pursued. If the problems you mutually identify occur mostly at home, then the goals should focus on the home. If the problems occur mostly at school, then your goals need to engage the school's teachers and staff. If you are seeing the patient in a primary care clinic, the treatment goals may include learning coping skills, developing new habits, or establishing care with a mental health practitioner. If you are seeing the patient in a hospital, the treatment goals usually address acute concerns, such as decreasing suicidality or improving mood.

Any good treatment goal can be achieved. It does no one a service to set unachievable goals. Unachievable goals are a species of magical thinking, the wish that simply thinking about something will make it happen. We may earnestly desire to play a highly competitive sport such as football (soccer) and represent our country in the World Cup, but no amount of training will ever help two middle-aged psychiatrists make the team. Similarly, it is foolish to set a goal that is truly impossible for a young person—whether because of age, developmental status, or physical or psychological characteristics—to achieve. It also does no one a service to set unexceptional goals. Unexceptional goals are a kind of everyday cruelty, the setting of a low bar to claim an unearned victory. We may not play a sport professionally, but we can (at least for now) tie our own shoes, so setting a treatment goal of shoelace tying would be insulting. The best goals are just a little bit out of reach of what seems possible; in our hypothetical case, our goal should be to improve our passing and shooting in games of pickup soccer/football. Pursuing similarly appropriate goals improves the lives of patients, caregivers, and clinicians because these goals expand our imagination for what is possible.

Writing about how setting the right goal can expand our imagination of the possible can seem too aspirational, so we remind you that goals must simultaneously be measurable. A treatment goal cannot be to "be healthier," "be less ill," or "have better behavior." Parents often say they want their children to be "good," which is a similarly unmeasurable goal. In our own example, a difficult-to-measure goal would be that we each "become a better footballer," whereas a measurable goal would be to "increase our passing accuracy from 50% to 75%." The treatment goals you set with patients also should be measurable so that you know when the patient is, or is not, achieving the goals you have agreed on.

Best Practices

One way to identify achievable and measurable goals is to personalize treatment goals to what is possible to achieve as reported in the medical literature. Several practice guidelines and treatment plans are available (e.g., Nurcombe 2014). In our work with young people, we prefer the practice parameters created and maintained by the American Academy of Child and Adolescent Psychiatry (AACAP). The parameters cover most of the major categories of mental illness that children and adolescents experience. The parameters were written by experts in the field and include information about etiology, diagnosis, treatment, and prognosis. All include specific recommendations that can be widely adopted. The practice parameters can be found online at www.jaacap.com/content/pracparam.

As of this writing, 59 practice parameters and guidelines are included in the AACAP library, far more than we can summarize here. Even if we could summarize them, they are dynamic documents, so we have dispersed some of the knowledge in the current practice parameters throughout this book, especially in the next three chapters. The American Psychiatric Association also has developed a set of clinical practice guidelines, but these are targeted to treatment in adult patients. Those guidelines of care may be found at http://psychiatryonline.org/guidelines. Table 14–1 provides some general advice for developing an initial treatment plan.

TABLE 14–1. Sequential steps for developing an initial treatment plan

1.   Identify your patient's initial treatment goal.

2.   Develop a therapeutic alliance with your patient.

3.   Clarify the relationship between the caregiver and your patient.

4.   Reach the most specific DSM-5 diagnosis.

5.   Write a hierarchical list of your patient's current problems.

6.   Rewrite the problem list into treatment goals.

7.   Identify measurable and achievable goals from the available evidence base.

8.   Customize the treatment for your patient's cultural background and available resources.

9.   Assign responsibility for each goal to a member of your patient's treatment team.

10.   Monitor the progress toward each goal.

11.   Revise the goals as your patient's situation changes.

Chapter 15

Initiating Psychosocial Interventions

When you assess and address a child or an adolescent's mental and behavioral health problems, you often direct caregivers to resources or interventions that they will deliver themselves. After all, most care for persons is delivered at home—where children are welcomed, fed, cleaned, taught, and nurtured. Motivated caregivers can implement evidence-supported care strategies that they learn from you or from handouts, books, websites, or videos you recommend. As noted in Chapter 2, "Meeting a Young Person Experiencing Mental Distress," such adjunctive therapy or bibliotherapy has been shown to be clinically effective in some situations. Pediatric primary care clinicians tend to be particularly skilled in the realm of offering psychosocial intervention advice because a key part of that professional role is offering parenting advice and anticipatory guidance.

This chapter contains selected highlights from among the psychosocial intervention strategies and tips we often describe for caregivers. Their inspiration comes from many different sources, including lessons from different lines of clinical research, general professional consensus, and personal experience (Chorpita and Daleiden 2009; Hilt 2024; Jellinek et al. 2002). This is not an exhaustive list of psychosocial strategies; but rather a few we like to share. These behavioral support strategies may be either sufficient on their own to resolve a mild concern or used to supplement specialist-delivered services.

Time-Out

Time-out is a strategy by which caregivers shape a young child's behavior through selective and temporary removal of that child's access to desired attention, activities, or other reinforcements following a behavioral transgression. This strategy works only for a child who experiences regular positive praise and attention from their caregiver because the child feels motivated to maintain that positive regard. The temporary removal of desired attention from a time-out can happen anywhere, not just via physically placing a child into a designated time-out area. It is often said that the length of a time-out should be about 1 minute for each year of age but adjusted for developmental level—for instance, time-outs for a developmentally delayed child should have shorter durations.

Although time-outs may be simple in concept, they are often difficult to implement. For example, parents commonly report having tried time-outs and found them ineffective before seeing a clinician. When a clinician analyzes how time-outs were conducted, it often becomes clear why a time-out strategy did not improve behavior. For instance, a time-out in which parent and child are yelling back and forth at each other through a closed door functions more like an attention reward "time-in" than a behavior-altering time-out. The following is a list of suggested parent tips for an effective time-out.

- To avoid confusion, set consistent limits.
- Focus on changing the priority misbehaviors rather than everything at once.
- After announcing the time-out, decline further verbal engagement until "time-in."
- Ensure that time-outs occur immediately after misbehavior instead of being delayed.
- Follow through if using warnings (e.g., "I'm going to count to three....").
- Minimize reinforcement of misbehavior with calm, quiet limit-setting.
- State when the time-out is over (the child does not determine this). Setting a timer can help.
- When the time-out is finished, simply resume business as usual or congratulate the child on regaining personal control. Then look for the next positive behavior to praise.
- For time-outs to help, give children far more positive attention than negative attention.

Social Media Pauses

Taking a *social media pause*, *fast*, or *vacation* allows people to take a step back from their social media accounts. After all, social media platforms profit by engaging the attention of users of all ages.

For young children, social media increases the risk of exposure to consumerism, pornography, and violence, so the Children's Online Privacy Protection Act sets a minimum age of 13 for social media platform use unless a parent offers verifiable consent. In research studies of 12-year-olds, the habitual use of social media is associated with changes in the amygdala and prefrontal cortex, increasing sensitivity to social rewards and punishments (Maza et al. 2023). Other researchers have found that early adolescent use predicts a subsequent decline in life satisfaction when social media is used during sensitive developmental windows (Orben et al. 2022). Although every child is different, we find that the risks of social media outweigh the benefits for children younger than age 16.

The benefits of social media, especially the ability to connect virtually with people with attributes and skills different from those of local peers, can be more beneficial for older adolescents. Adolescents, like adults, can form community over social media platforms and create opportunities that enhance their lives.

However, a growing body of evidence suggests that adolescents, like adults, suffer when they spend excessive time on social media platforms. In a large cohort study, researchers found that adolescents ages 12–15 who spent 3 hours or more daily on social media doubled their risk of negative mental health outcomes (Riehm et al. 2019).

Fortunately, the effects work in the opposite direction as well: decreasing the use of social media or taking a 4-week pause are both associated with improved mental well-being (Allcott et al. 2020; Hunt et al. 2018). If a child, adolescent, or caregiver finds themselves spending more time than anticipated on social media, experiencing negative cognitions and emotions with social media use, or missing in-person events because of social media use, it can be helpful to take a pause.

The rules are different for each social media platform, but settings are typically available that allow a child, adolescent, or caregiver to pause or silence a social media account. Look for settings to deactivate, delete, or disable an account. The settings are often difficult to access, so try looking online for current ways to pause social media. The following is a list of parent tips for successful use of social media.

- Delay social media use by children and adolescents, ideally until age 16 or later.
- Turn on screen time settings for commonly used devices and apps to track usage.
- Set (and follow) goals for how much time to spend on social media.
- Enable nightly do not disturb settings to enable sleep.
- Turn on settings that allow caregivers to monitor social media use for younger and more vulnerable users.
- Turn off notifications.
- Engage children and adolescents in discussion about which social media platforms encourage community and well-being.
- Delete social media that discourages community and well-being.
- Encourage adolescents to take regular social media vacations, especially over school and cultural holidays.
- Develop a set of expectations for social media use that children, parents, and adolescents can follow together, such as not using devices during meals and addressing familial conflicts in person. Determine whether and how to share photos and videos as part of a family media plan, which establishes boundaries.
- Take a weekly holiday from social media as a family.
- Report inappropriate social media behavior such as cyberbullying and harassment.

Special Time

Special time is a way for a caregiver and young child to reestablish the enjoyment of each other's company. Sometimes this reestablishment of positive caregiver-child interactions alone will be able to resolve a chronic behavior problem. Special time also can be referred to as *child-directed play* because it emphasizes that parents spend that time following their child's lead and attending to what the child can do. The following is a list of parent tips for successful use of special time.

- Commit to setting aside a regular time to try this with your child. Daily is best, but two or three times a week consistently also works.

- Select the time of day, labeling it as something like *our play time*, *our calendar time*, or *our special time*.
- Choose a time short enough that it can happen reliably, usually 15–30 minutes.
- Once this one-on-one time is planned, ensure that it happens no matter how good or bad the day was.
- Allow the child to pick the activity, which must be something you do not actively dislike and that does not involve spending money or completing a chore.
- Follow the child's lead during play, resisting urges to tell them what to do.
- End on time; using a timer may help. Remind the child when the next special time will be.
- If the child refuses at first, explain that you will just sit with them for their special time.
- Expect greater success if you as a caregiver separately get your own special or nurturing times too.

Functional Analysis (of Behavior)

Functional analysis is a general strategy for resolving a recurrent problem behavior. Functional analysis is most often cited as a treatment for a child with developmental impairments or a limited verbal capacity, but its principles apply to any child. The objective is to first identify *why* a behavior keeps recurring and then intelligently devise a plan to prevent future repetitions.

For instance, imagine a young child throws tantrums during trips to stores. When a clinician helps to analyze the behavior's function, the child's caregiver realizes he has been giving the child candy to halt the tantrums, which for the child functionally serves to reward the behavior and encourage it to happen again. If the caregiver chooses to stop delivering these unintentional rewards, the tantrum behavior would be theorized to decrease, although usually after a temporary increase in the behavior while the child tests out the flexibility of the new rules (an *extinction burst*). Alternatively, the caregiver may focus on avoiding reexposing the child to a recognized behavior trigger, such as no longer bringing the child into a store's candy aisle. The following is a list of tips for performing a functional analysis of behavior (Hanley et al. 2003; Hilt 2024).

1. Identify the behavior.

   • Determine the character, timing (especially what happens right before and after), frequency, and duration of the behavior.

2. Analyze and hypothesize about the behavior's function.

   • Achieve a goal: This might include escaping an undesired situation, avoiding a transition, acquiring attention, or getting access to desired things.
   • Communicate: Maladaptive behavior may communicate physical or emotional discomfort.
   • If no function is clear, other causes such as medical or psychiatric disorders, medication side effects, and sleep deprivation become more likely.

3. Make a change, usually by changing something in the environment.

   • Remove future reinforcements for the maladaptive behavior (attention or other gains).
   • Avoid known behavioral triggers.
   • Modify task demands to be appropriate for the child's developmental stage and language ability.
   • Reinforce positive behaviors with attention and praise.
   • Enhance communication (e.g., help a nonverbal child use pictures to communicate).
   • Clarify any unclear expectations—show or follow a daily schedule, prepare the child for transitions.
   • Allow the child access to escapes when they are overwhelmed (specified amount of time in a calm, quiet place).

4. Analyze whether the interventions worked, and, if not, repeat the process.

   • Look for improvements in the behavior's timing, character, frequency, and duration.

Behavioral Activation

Behavioral activation is a way to help a young person reengage with other people. When a young person is sad or worried, they are less likely to engage in the activities they typically enjoy, and this withdrawal from otherwise pleasurable activities deepens isolation and lowers mood. Therefore, despite areas of difference, most cognitive-behavioral therapies for depression and anxiety seek behavioral activation. After all, the path to recovery from depression and anxiety does not begin with spending all your time alone and unproductive. Increases in youth depression and anxiety, coupled with pandemic-era school and social lockdowns, emphasize how individual isolation can result in population-wide failures.

In behavioral activation, a person pushes to more regularly do things that they find pleasurable or that serve their goals. If they can accomplish this behavioral activation, their symptoms usually improve. The challenge is to create the necessary motivation when feeling depressed or anxious. The following is a list of tips for succeeding with behavioral activation.

- Identify activities that you (not others) would find motivating or rewarding. Work on developing a variety of options because repetitively doing the same thing can get boring.
- Refine the list to things that can be measured as completed rather than relatively vague goals that you cannot determine have been completed.
- Rank the activities in order from those that would be easier to complete to those that would be more difficult to complete.
- Start by selecting something easy to accomplish to get started, and work your way up the list from there.
- Let others know your plans to increase your activities, and enlist their help in motivating you further.

Confronting Bullying

For years, it has been recognized that bullying is both common and harmful for both the victim and the perpetrator. If you notice a relatively sudden change in a child's mood, behavior, sleep, or body symptoms or any sudden change in social or academic functioning, then you should consider the possibility the child is being bullied.

If bullying is discovered, it is often challenging for an adult to know how to respond. The following is a list of tips for how to respond to bullying (Buxton et al. 2013; Hilt 2024).

1. Detect
   - Ask the child, *"I know kids sometimes get picked on or bullied. Have you ever seen this happen? Has this ever happened to you?"*
   - If the child says no but you still suspect bullying, have caregivers ask teachers about bullying and/or review the child's social media accounts.

2. Educate
   - Let children know that bullying is unacceptable and that if they encounter bullying, you will help them respond.

3. Plan
   - Coach the child to avoid places where bullying happens.
   - Teach the child to walk away when bullying occurs and tell a trusted adult who can be accessed quickly.
   - Instruct a child to stay near adults—most bullying happens when no adults are around.
   - If a child feels that they can confront the bully, teach them to say, in a calm, clear voice, to stop the behavior, that "bullying is not OK."
   - Note that if the child is comfortable deflating situations with humor, they may use humor to challenge the bullying.
   - Encourage the child to ask their peers for their support and ideas.
   - Ensure that caregivers communicate the problem to the child's school and other families, jointly devising solutions.

4. Support
   - Tell caregivers to encourage participation in prosocial activities to build peer networks, enhance social skills, and gain confidence.

Additional information is available on websites such as www.stopbullying.gov.

Sleep Hygiene

Sleep hygiene is a good idea for anyone, but especially for young people. Insomnia is a common problem among children and adolescents. Most sleep problems can be resolved by changing habits and routines that affect sleep, what clinicians call *good sleep hygiene*. For instance, when sleep is a problem, it can work wonders to coach parents and youth around eliminating access to what we might label the *sleep prevention device* (a smartphone) in the bedroom certain hours of the day. The following is a list of parent tips for how to improve sleep hygiene (Hilt 2024; Mindell and Owens 2009).

- Maintain consistent bedtimes and wake times every day of the week.
- Maintain a routine of pre-sleep activities (e.g., read a book, brush teeth).
- Avoid having the child spend non-sleep time in or on their bed (i.e., beds are for sleep).
- Ensure that the bedroom is cool and quiet.
- Avoid high-stimulation activities (television, video games, texting friends, or exercise) just before bed or during awakenings.
- Do not keep video games, televisions, computers, or smartphones in a child's bedroom.
- Have the child exercise earlier in the day.
- Avoid caffeine in the afternoons and evenings; caffeine can cause shallow sleep or frequent awakenings.
- If a child or an adolescent is awake in bed and unable to sleep, have them get out of bed for a low-stimulation activity (e.g., reading), then return 20–30 minutes later. This keeps the bed from becoming associated with sleeplessness.
- Encourage children and adolescents to discuss any worries with a caregiver before bed rather than ruminating later.
- Ensure that children go to bed drowsy but still awake. Falling asleep in other places forms habits that are difficult to break.
- Use security objects at bedtime for a young child who needs a transitional object to feel safe and secure when a caregiver is not present.
- When checking on a young child at night, aim to only briefly reassure the child that you are present and that they are OK.
- Avoid afternoon naps for all but the very young because they often interfere with nighttime sleep.
- If a child or an adolescent is still having difficulties sleeping, keep a sleep diary to help you track their naps, sleep times, and activities to identify patterns.

Gratitude Exercises

Positive psychology examines evidence-based methods for human flourishing, including cognitive exercises (e.g., imagining your best possible self), behavioral exercises (e.g., performing acts of kindness), relational practices (e.g., participating in a faith community), and workbooks to achieve forgiveness or similar emotional states (VanderWeele 2020). Although most of the available research has been conducted among adults, many of these activities can be adapted and recommended for children and adolescents.

For example, gratitude exercises are cognitive actions that can improve psychological well-being (Davis et al. 2016) and will likely benefit any child or adolescent. A family could end the day with gratitude exercises by, say, asking a child before they sleep to recall three good things from the day. A parent could establish a weekly practice of writing down five things about a child or adolescent they are grateful for and slipping it into their school lunch box on Mondays. Gratitude exercises should not be paired with criticism or feedback, as in the so-called compliment sandwich but rather should stand alone as an opportunity to practice gratitude as a cognitive state. So a college student could write down five things they are grateful for, instead of their struggles, each Saturday and email them home. Over time, such exercises help people focus on their blessings instead of their burdens and instill a spirit of gratitude (Emmons and McCullough 2003).

Chapter 16

Starting a Psychotherapy

Every treatment plan for a young person with a mental disorder includes the formation of a therapeutic alliance with you as the clinician and psychoeducation about diagnosis, treatment, and prognosis. The most effective treatment plan usually includes some form of psychotherapy. There are many evidence-based textbooks that can teach more advanced psychotherapy techniques for working with children and adolescents (e.g., Christophersen and VanScoyoc 2013; Kendall 2012; Weisz and Kazdin 2010). These psychotherapy skills are typically learned during training programs when senior clinicians supervise trainees. Although we recommend these texts and psychotherapy training to everyone who regularly works with children and adolescents, in this chapter we introduce different kinds of psychotherapy, discuss how to select a particular psychotherapy, and explain how to engage a child and their caregivers in psychotherapy.

Psychotherapy is an important treatment strategy for young people for many reasons. It is almost always the safest treatment option we can offer and has the least potential for adverse effects. Also, for specific problems, such as disruptive behavior or suicidality, it has shown superior efficacy over psychotropic medication interventions. In addition, the psychotherapy literature has shown that when a person attributes a behavioral change to their own efforts, the change is more enduring than a behavioral change they attribute to an external source, such as a medication (Alarcón and Frank 2011).

However, the changes that result from psychotherapy generally are not immediate—we expect it to take a month or two of regular sessions before a child or an adolescent begins to manifest the benefits of psychotherapy. This delay is part of the reason why it is important to stratify the severity of a young person's mental distress. If a child or an adolescent is having moderate to severe difficulties, our preferred treatment plan is more likely to include a combination of psychotherapy and medication, when a medication is appropriate for their diagnosis, to encourage the most rapid and reliable results. For young people who have mild mental health difficulties, our treatment plans typically begin with psychotherapy alone. Of course, these are broad generalizations, and many exceptions exist. For instance, even with severe oppositional defiant disorder, we prefer to start treatment with behavior management training instead of psychotropic medications. In contrast, it is clinically reasonable to initiate treatment for severe attention-deficit/hyperactivity disorder with stimulant medications alone.

If you decide to recommend psychotherapy, it can be difficult to know which psychotherapy to recommend because a growing number of validated psychotherapies can be delivered to children. A simple heuristic is to match a maladaptive stress response to a type of therapy (Table 16–1).

Next, you can select a more specific psychotherapy by looking at resources like those maintained by the U.S. Substance Abuse and Mental Health Services Administration. For example, its website (www.samhsa.gov/resource-search/ebp) lists hundreds of different research evidence–based psychotherapies and treatment approaches for young people with mental health and substance use challenges. Fortunately, even though these therapies have significant differences, they are often variations on a small number of themes. For example, TF-CBT seems like a confusing acronym, but it is a trauma-focused version of cognitive-behavioral therapy, a widely practiced evidence-based psychotherapy.

Even after you identify the appropriate psychotherapy for a particular child or adolescent, it can be difficult to engage a young person and their caregivers in the therapy. Meta-analyses show that between 25% and 75% of children and adolescents in mental health treatment prematurely discontinue (de Haan et al. 2013), a finding that illustrates the challenges of delivering treatment. Barriers to engagement in psychotherapy include stigma, ambivalence about behavior change, doubts about the efficacy of psychotherapy, the time investment it requires, or financial barriers. You can help by communicating appropriate expectations for psychotherapy with a patient and their caregivers, informing them of the efficacy of psychotherapy, the delayed response, and its enduring benefits.

How else can you engage a patient and their caregivers in psychotherapy?

TABLE 16–1. Psychotherapy families to consider

Maladaptive response	Psychotherapy family
Justifications	Cognitive
Defenses	Psychodynamic
Relationships	Family
Experiences	Experiential
Habits	Behavioral

- Explain the diagnosis in a way that the patient and their caregivers can fully understand.
- Explain the rationale for the psychotherapy treatment plan (e.g., it is the safest or most effective approach).
- Briefly describe what the recommended psychotherapy experience would be like.
- Ask whether they have any concerns about the approach and address them.
- Provide the family with a list of recommended clinicians.
- Follow up with the family to address any problems that arise.

This last follow-up step is particularly important because families often get discouraged if they run into an insurance coverage restriction or have trouble finding an available clinician. There is often a relative shortage of skilled therapists available to see young people with mental health care needs, so it takes time and tenacity for families to connect with care. Discussing what happened with the referral provides you an opportunity to amend the care plan. In general, referrals are most successful when you can match a patient and their caregiver with a therapist with whom they form a therapeutic alliance (Roos and Werbart 2013).

After all, the heart of all psychiatric treatments is the therapeutic alliance you establish when a patient identifies treatment goals and you ally yourself with the patient as they pursue those goals. You form an alliance between yourself and your patient with the goal of mobilizing healing forces within your patient by psychological means. Your ability to form these alliances profoundly influences the efficacy of your work for the patient as well as your satisfaction with this work (Summers and Barber 2003). To assist you, we have prepared descriptions of different types of psychotherapy that are commonly considered with children and adolescents and a list of conditions for which their use has been validated as effective by research (Table 16–2).

TABLE 16–2. Commonly recommended child and adolescent psychotherapies

Therapy	General description	Typical indications
Cognitive-behavioral therapy (CBT)	Teaches patients how to correct illness-related cognitive errors in thinking (e.g., the depressed patient thinking "nothing ever goes right for me") and coaches and encourages patients to try out different behaviors (i.e., behavior activation), both of which lead to changes in how the person feels. Assigning practice and trials between sessions is a core feature. Desensitization via supported exposure to one's fears is typically used for anxiety.	Anxiety disorders (all) Depressive disorders Oppositional defiant disorder Eating disorders Substance use disorders
Trauma-focused CBT	Most cited version of trauma therapy in children. Starts with building therapeutic support and educating about PTSD. Like other successful trauma therapies, treatment requires patients to face their own trauma narrative to desensitize, reduce pathological avoidance, and reduce the trauma memory's control over their future.	PTSD
Dialectical behavior therapy	Very specialized version of CBT; requires attending skills groups (to teach problem-solving, emotional regulation, distress tolerance, and interpersonal effectiveness skills) and attending individual therapy sessions. Mindfulness and meditative exercises are often used to assist. Uniquely helpful for treatment-resistant, chronically suicidal patients. Most supportive research is with adults.	Chronic and significant suicidality and self-harm

TABLE 16–2. Commonly recommended child and adolescent psychotherapies *(continued)*

Therapy	General description	Typical indications
Family therapy	Many different styles and approaches, but all focus on the family relationship or interaction patterns that cause dysfunction and help the family system to amend that pattern (rather than identifying a mental health diagnosis to treat or saying that the problem resides within an individual).	Eating disorders Conduct disorder Depressive disorders Substance use disorders
Group therapy	Addresses problems with interaction patterns, as in family therapy, while providing more disorder-specific support within a group of strangers having similar challenges. Peer-based learning can be uniquely effective. Therapists must steer group members away from inadvertently teaching unhealthy behaviors.	Anxiety disorders
Behavior management training	General term for programs teaching and encouraging skillful parent or caregiver responses to challenging child behaviors. Positive interaction time between the parent and the child is encouraged because it must accompany behavior management steps to work. Changing caregiver behaviors is key rather than changing the child through individual therapy sessions. Also known as *parent management training*.	Oppositional defiant disorder Conduct disorder

TABLE 16–2. Commonly recommended child and adolescent psychotherapies (*continued*)

Therapy	General description	Typical indications
Applied behavior analysis	One-on-one specialized intensive behavior management training that gradually teaches socially normative behaviors via small achievable elements, with each element reinforced by a reward (such as rewarding the child making any "h" sound as a step in teaching the use of "hello"). Highly resource intensive in terms of the required therapist hours and continuous treatment planning.	Autism spectrum disorder
Social skills training	Variety of class-based, group, and one-on-one techniques for teaching basic behavioral and cognitive skills, reinforcing prosocial behaviors, and teaching social problem-solving. More potent when delivered in a group rather than a one-on-one setting because of peer-learning influences.	Oppositional defiant disorder ADHD Autism spectrum disorder
Relaxation training	Biofeedback, deep breathing, progressive muscle relaxation, and mindfulness are examples of strategies used to increase mind-body awareness and the ability to electively calm the heights of emotional reactions. Must be practiced when not in crisis to develop the skills needed in times of crisis.	Anxiety disorders Depressive disorders

TABLE 16–2. Commonly recommended child and adolescent psychotherapies (*continued*)

Therapy	General description	Typical indications
Motivational interviewing	Therapeutic interaction regarding health behavior(s) around which a patient needs to change but has significant reluctance to change. Nonconfrontationally and nonjudgmentally helps patients to state their own reasons for changing, to resolve their own ambivalence, and to state what actions they could take to change. Most supportive research is with adults.	Substance use disorders

Chapter 17

Initiating Medications and Monitoring for Adverse Effects

Clinicians commonly prescribe psychotropic medications to children and adolescents. For example, in national cross-sectional studies of ambulatory care, more than 6% of surveyed adolescents in the United States reported using a psychotropic medication in the past month, and nearly 8% of all primary care visits in 2015 involved youth being prescribed stimulant medications (Girand et al. 2020; Jonas et al. 2013; Pringsheim et al. 2019). This relatively widespread use of psychotropic medications means that caregivers have come to expect primary care clinicians, not just mental health specialists, to consider prescribing medication for a child or an adolescent with a mental illness.

When should a clinician prescribe a psychotropic medication? Not every child with depression, anxiety, or attention-deficit/hyperactivity disorder (ADHD) needs to receive a medication, regardless of whether it fits an approved or research-supported indication. Because psychiatric medications can cause adverse effects, you must, at a minimum, believe that the potential benefit of psychotropic medication exceeds the potential risks your patient may experience. For instance, if a child has a relatively mild case of depression, psychotherapy alone is usually sufficient and the most appropriate way to help, and its use does not introduce the risk of adverse medical effects. If a child or an adolescent's depression is more severe or persistent, it makes more sense clinically to use a selective serotonin reuptake inhibitor (SSRI) combined with psychotherapy to achieve a more rapid rate of recovery (e.g., Emslie et al. 2010).

As a rule of thumb, if a child or an adolescent has a moderate to severe range of symptoms and an evidence-based psychotropic medication is available, we usually prescribe the medication at the same time we initiate the appropriate psychosocial interventions. For a child or an adolescent with milder symptoms, we generally recommend starting treatment with psychotherapy, family, or environmental interventions alone. Patients with mild symptoms but persistent dysfunction become stronger candidates for a medication treatment when nonmedication strategies prove ineffective.

When approaching the decision about what to prescribe, we advise following evidence-based principles. Although we appreciate the wisdom of experienced clinicians and the insights reported in case series, these are small, unstandardized accounts. Whenever possible, we base our prescribing decisions on evidence generated from controlled trials conducted among children and adolescents. We recommend that clinicians who frequently prescribe psychotropic medications to children and adolescents read the evidence-based systematic reviews published in the *Cochrane Database of Systematic Reviews*, the "Clinical Practice Guidelines" published by the American Academy of Child and Adolescent Psychiatry, or a high-quality textbook (e.g., Dulcan 2022; McVoy and Findling 2017).

When such evidence is unavailable, we find that research on adult mental health medication is informative but in need of translation before we can use the medication for children and adolescents. Children and adolescents are not little adults who will respond to little doses. For example, tricyclic antidepressants are effective in the treatment of depression in adults, but controlled trials have found that they are no better than placebo in the treatment of depression in children and are of marginal utility for treating depression in adolescents (Hazell and Mirzaie 2013; Murphy et al. 2021). A result from the literature on adult mental health therefore must be replicated in children and adolescents before it can be reliably followed.

However, appropriate evidence-based care does not mean limiting your prescriptions to only those medications approved for children and adolescents by a regulatory agency such as the FDA. Across pediatric health care, about half of all prescribed medications lack an age-matched pediatric regulatory approval—an issue that is not unique to mental health care (Yackey et al. 2019). This regulatory discrepancy occurs largely because the process of obtaining regulatory approval is a long and expensive endeavor that requires a vested party (usually the manufacturer). Even without a regulator's approval, rigorous research may exist to support a particular use of medication. The likelihood of being prescribed medications on-label versus off-label depends on many factors, like the medication itself, the treatment indication, the age of the child, and the location of care (Braüner et al. 2016).

Some of the key questions we ask ourselves before prescribing any medication include the following:

- Diagnosis—does the child have an evidence-based medication indication?
- Age—how does the child's age change your risk-benefit analysis?
- Severity—how rapid of a treatment response is needed?
- History—what has already been tried, and how effective was it?
- Preferences—are there strong patient or caregiver opinions about the use of medication?
- Risks—does the medication present any unacceptable risks relative to the treatment goal?

When patients and caregivers are struggling, clinicians can feel pressured to use medications outside of evidence-based indications. We prefer to resist these demands and limit the prescription of psychotropic medications to the indications for which sound evidence exists. For instance, to prescribe methylphenidate for a child whose poor school performance is not due to ADHD but rather is due to a learning disability, anxiety, social distractions, or depression may be ineffective and may delay the use of more appropriate interventions. Similarly, antipsychotics may reduce the severity of nonspecific aggression, but they are unlikely to address the underlying causes of youth aggression and may unnecessarily introduce major adverse effects.

Tables 17–1 to 17–5 include only those psychotropic medications with an evidence base from randomized controlled trials for use with young people. We use these tables as a quick reference point of research-supported medications rather than an exhaustive reference and review of all information available. The age ranges of the listed FDA approvals do not necessarily reflect the age ranges for which these medications are clinically appropriate or effective.

Older antipsychotic medications with long-standing FDA approvals for use in young people include haloperidol (≥3 years old) for severe aggression and Tourette's disorder, pimozide (≥12 years old) for Tourette's disorder, chlorprom-

TABLE 17–1. ADHD: short-acting evidence-based stimulant medications

Medication name	Stimulant class	Duration (hours)	Usual 6- to 10-year-old starting dosages (mg)	Available doses (mg tablets)	FDA maximum daily dose (mg; approval ages)	Editorial comments
Methylphenidate (Ritalin, Methylin)	Methylphenidate	4–6	5 bid (2.5 if 3–5 years)	5, 10, 20	60 (≥6)	May have fewer side effects than dextroamphetamine; better evidence for very young children
Dexmethylphenidate (Focalin)	Methylphenidate	4–6	2.5 bid (1.25 if 3–5 years)	2.5, 5, 10	20 (≥6)	Racemic isomer, so has twice the mg:mg potency of methylphenidate

TABLE 17–1. ADHD: short-acting evidence-based stimulant medications *(continued)*

Medication name	Stimulant class	Duration (hours)	Usual 6- to 10-year-old starting dosages (mg)	Available doses (mg tablets)	FDA maximum daily dose (mg; approval ages)	Editorial comments
Dextroamphetamine (Dexedrine, Dextrostat, ProCentra, Zenzedi)	Dextroamphetamine	4–6	2.5 bid (1.25 if 3–5 years)	2.5, 5, 7.5, 10, 20, 30	40 (≥3)	Tends to have longer duration than methylphenidate; slightly more side effects
Amphetamine salt combination (Adderall)	Dextroamphetamine	4–6	2.5 bid (1.25 if 3–5 years)	5, 7.5, 10, 12.5, 15, 20, 30	40 (≥3)	Tends to have longer duration than methylphenidate; slightly more side effects
D- and L-amphetamine sulfate (Evekeo)	Dextroamphetamine	4–6	2.5 bid (1.25 if 3–5 years)	5, 10, 15, 20	40 (≥3)	Oral disintegrating tablet form available

TABLE 17–2. ADHD: long-acting evidence-based stimulant medications

Medication name	Stimulant class	Duration (hours)	Usual 6- to 10-year-old starting dosages (mg)	Available doses	FDA maximum daily dose (mg; approval ages)	Editorial comments
Methylphenidate ER/SR (Metadate ER)	Methylphenidate	4–8	10 qam	10, 20 mg tablets	60 (≥6)	Uses a wax matrix for delivery; variable duration of action
OROS methylphenidate (Concerta)	Methylphenidate	10–12	18 qam	18, 27, 36, 54 mg capsules	72 (≥6)	Osmotic release capsule; cannot be cut or crushed
Methylphenidate XR oral suspension (Quillivant XR)	Methylphenidate	Up to 8	10 qam	5 mg/mL liquid	60 (≥6)	Microsuspension yields an ER liquid
Methylphenidate XR microcoated chewable (Quillichew ER)	Methylphenidate	~8	10 qam	20, 30, 40 mg tablets	60 (≥6)	Chewable tablets, scored

TABLE 17–2. ADHD: long-acting evidence-based stimulant medications (*continued*)

Medication name	Stimulant class	Duration (hours)	Usual 6- to 10-year-old starting dosages (mg)	Available doses	FDA maximum daily dose (mg; approval ages)	Editorial comments
Methylphenidate XR; 30% IR, 70% ER (Metadate CD)	Methylphenidate	8–10	10 qam	10, 20, 30, 40, 50, 60 mg capsules	60 (≥6)	Beads in capsule, more afternoon release, can be sprinkled on food
Methylphenidate XR; 40% IR, 60% ER (Aptensio XR)	Methylphenidate	~10	10 qam	10, 15, 20, 30, 40, 50, 60 mg capsules	60 (≥6)	Beads in capsule, more afternoon release, can be sprinkled on food
Methylphenidate XR; 50% IR, 50% ER (Ritalin LA)	Methylphenidate	~8	10 qam	10, 20, 30, 40 mg capsules	60 (≥6)	Beads in capsule can be sprinkled on food

TABLE 17–2. ADHD: long-acting evidence-based stimulant medications (*continued*)

Medication name	Stimulant class	Duration (hours)	Usual 6- to 10-year-old starting dosages (mg)	Available doses	FDA maximum daily dose (mg; approval ages)	Editorial comments
Dexmethylphenidate XR (Focalin XR)	Methylphenidate	10–12	5 qam	5, 10, 15, 20 mg capsules	30 (≥6)	Beads in capsule are a racemic isomer of methylphenidate, so twice the mg potency
Methylphenidate patch (Daytrana)	Methylphenidate	3–5 hours after patch removal	10 qam	10, 15, 20, 30 mg patch	30 (≥6)	Site rash problems; slow morning startup of effects; works until removed

TABLE 17–2. ADHD: long-acting evidence-based stimulant medications (*continued*)

Medication name	Stimulant class	Duration (hours)	Usual 6- to 10-year-old starting dosages (mg)	Available doses	FDA maximum daily dose (mg; approval ages)	Editorial comments
Methylphenidate overnight delay (Jornay PM)	Methylphenidate	12 hours after 10-hour delay	20 qpm	20, 40, 60, 80, 100 mg capsules	100 (≥6)	Beads in capsule, give at bedtime for morning release
Methylphenidate oral disintegrating (Cotempla XR-ODT)	Methylphenidate	10–12	17.3 qam	8.6, 17.3, 25.9 mg tablets	51.8 (≥6)	Tablet needs to disintegrate on tongue without crushing or chewing
Amphetamine mixed salt combo XR (Adderall XR)	Dextroamphetamine	8–12	5 qd	5, 10, 15, 20, 25, 30 mg capsules	30 (≥6)	Generic available; beads in capsule can be sprinkled on food

TABLE 17–2. ADHD: long-acting evidence-based stimulant medications (*continued*)

Medication name	Stimulant class	Duration (hours)	Usual 6- to 10-year-old starting dosages (mg)	Available doses	FDA maximum daily dose (mg; approval ages)	Editorial comments
Amphetamine d- and l- salt combo XR (Adzenys ODT)	Dextroamphetamine	8–12	6.3 qd	3.1, 6.3, 9.4, 12.5, 15.7, 18.8 mg tablets	18.8 (6–12)	Oral disintegrating tablet; about 2 times the potency of the same mg amount of Adderall XR
Amphetamine salt combo XR triple bead (Mydayis)	Dextroamphetamine	16	12.5 qam	12.5, 25, 37.5, 50 mg capsules	25 (13–17)	Three-bead design means very long delivery; not approved for children younger than 13

TABLE 17–2. ADHD: long-acting evidence-based stimulant medications *(continued)*

Medication name	Stimulant class	Duration (hours)	Usual 6- to 10-year-old starting dosages (mg)	Available doses	FDA maximum daily dose (mg; approval ages)	Editorial comments
Lisdexamfetamine (Vyvanse)	Dextroamphetamine	~10	30 qd	20, 30, 40, 50, 60, 70 mg capsules	70 (≥6)	Conversion ratio from dextroamphetamine not well established; gastro-intestinal bioactivation
Dextroamphetamine ER (Dexedrine Spansule)	Dextroamphetamine	8–10	5 qam	5, 10, 15 mg capsules	40 (≥6)	Beads in capsule can be sprinkled on food
Dextroamphetamine oral suspension (Dyanavel XR)	Dextroamphetamine	8–12	2.5 to 5 qam	2.5 mg/mL suspension	20 (≥6)	Delayed release suspension

Note. ER=extended release; IR=immediate release; OROS=osmotic controlled-release oral delivery system; SR=sustained release; XR=extended release.

TABLE 17–3. ADHD: nonstimulant evidence-based medications

Medication name	Half-life (hours)	Medication type	Usual starting dosages	Available doses (mg)	FDA maximum daily dose (approval ages)	Editorial comments
Atomoxetine (Strattera)	5	Norepinephrine reuptake inhibitor	0.5 mg/kg once a day then 1.2 mg/kg/day after 1 week	10, 18, 25, 40, 60, 80, 100 capsules	100 mg or 1.4 mg/kg, whichever is less (≥6)	Side effect risks the same as with SSRIs (e.g., suicidality warning); cytochrome P450 2D6 metabolism; about 50% respond
Viloxazine (Qelbree)	7	Norepinephrine reuptake inhibitor	100 mg qd	100, 150, 200 capsules	400 mg (≥6)	Very similar effects and risks as atomoxetine; can open capsule onto food
Clonidine (Catapres)	12.5	Central-acting α_2-agonist	0.05 mg bid	0.1, 0.2, 0.3, 0.4 tablets	0.4 mg	Dosing at bedtime may help manage sedation effects

TABLE 17–3. ADHD: nonstimulant evidence-based medications *(continued)*

Medication name	Half-life (hours)	Medication type	Usual starting dosages	Available doses (mg)	FDA maximum daily dose (approval ages)	Editorial comments
Clonidine XR (Kapvay)	12.5	Central-acting α_2-agonist	0.1 mg qd	0.1, 0.2, 0.3, 0.4 tablets	0.4 mg ($\geq$6)	Difference is a reduced peak blood level relative to the IR form
Guanfacine (Tenex)	16	Central-acting α_2-agonist	1 mg qd	1, 2, 3, 4 tablets	4 mg	Dosing at bedtime may help manage sedation effects
Guanfacine XR (Intuniv)	18	Central-acting α_2-agonist	1 mg qd	0.1, 0.2, 0.3, 0.4 tablets	7 mg ($\geq$6)	Difference is a reduced peak blood level relative to the IR form

Note. IR=immediate release; SSRI=selective serotonin reuptake inhibitor; XR=extended release. Unlike stimulants, these medications may take up to a month to generate their full efficacy in the treatment of ADHD in children and adolescents. Stimulants are considered the first-line treatment option.

TABLE 17–4. Depressive and anxiety disorders: evidence-based medications

Medication name	Half-life	Usual teenage starting dosage (mg)	FDA maximum daily doses (approval ages)	Available doses (mg)	Conditions with RCT support	Editorial comments
Fluoxetine (Prozac)	4–6 days	10 qam	60 mg (≥7 OCD, ≥8 MDD)	10, 20, 40 capsules	OCD, MDD, GAD, SAD, SOC	First-line treatment for both depression and anxiety; long half-life reduces side effects from missed doses
Sertraline (Zoloft)	27 hours	50 qam	200 mg (≥6 OCD)	25, 50, 100 tablets	OCD, MDD, GAD, SAD, SOC	First-line treatment for anxiety; easy to use small doses (i.e., half of a 25-mg tablet)
Citalopram (Celexa)	35 hours	20 qam	40 mg in adults (not approved for children)	10, 20, 40 tablets	MDD, OCD	Very few medication interactions
Escitalopram (Lexapro)	29.5 hours	10 qam	20 mg (≥12 MDD)	5, 10, 20 tablets	MDD	Racemic isomer of citalopram; very few medication interactions

TABLE 17–4. Depressive and anxiety disorders: evidence-based medications *(continued)*

Medication name	Half-life	Usual teenage starting dosage (mg)	FDA maximum daily doses (approval ages)	Available doses (mg)	Conditions with RCT support	Editorial comments
Fluvoxamine (Luvox)	16 hours	25 qam	300 mg (≥8 OCD)	25, 50, 100 tablets	OCD, GAD, SOC, SAD	Often more side effects than other SSRIs; many medication interactions; thus, not a first-line option
Paroxetine (Paxil)	18 hours	20 qam	40 mg in adults (not approved for children)	10, 20, 30, 40 tablets	SOC	Mixed evidence; not preferred for child depression
Clomipramine (Anafranil)	32 hours	25 qam or qhs	200 mg or 3 mg/kg (≥10 OCD)	25, 50, 75 capsules	OCD	Tricyclic, used for treatment-resistant OCD; not a first-line option because of greater adverse effects than with SSRIs

TABLE 17–4. Depressive and anxiety disorders: evidence-based medications (*continued*)

Medication name	Half-life	Usual teenage starting dosage (mg)	FDA maximum daily doses (approval ages)	Available doses (mg)	Conditions with RCT support	Editorial comments
Duloxetine (Cymbalta)	12 hours	30 qd	120 mg (≥7 GAD)	20, 30, 60 capsules	GAD	SNRI; may have more adverse effects than SSRIs
Venlafaxine ER (Effexor ER)	5 (and 11 for active metabolite) hours	37.5 qd	225 mg in adults (not approved for children)	37.5, 75, 150 tablets or capsules	MDD	SNRI; more adverse effects than SSRIs

Note. ER=extended release; GAD=generalized anxiety disorder; MDD=major depressive disorder; RCT=randomized controlled trial; SAD=separation anxiety disorder; SNRI=serotonin-norepinephrine reuptake inhibitor; SOC=social anxiety disorder; SSRI=selective serotonin reuptake inhibitor.

TABLE 17–5. Bipolar and psychotic disorders: evidence-based medications

Medication name	Half-life (hours)	Usual teenage starting dosage (mg)	FDA maximum daily doses (mg; approval ages)	Available doses (mg)	Conditions with RCT support	Editorial comments
Risperidone (Risperdal)	17	0.5 qd	6 (≥13 schizophrenia, ≥10 bipolar mania, ≥5 autism irritability)	0.25, 0.5, 1, 2, 3, 4 tablets	Schizophrenia, bipolar mania, autism, Tourette's disorder	Extensively studied in children; has relatively consistent and rapid effects; extra risk of prolactinemia
Aripiprazole (Abilify)	75	2 qd	30 (≥13 schizophrenia, ≥10 bipolar mania, ≥6 autism irritability, ≥6 Tourette's disorder)	2, 5, 10, 15, 20 tablets	Schizophrenia, bipolar mania, autism, Tourette's disorder	Mixed agonist/antagonist at dopamine receptor D_2; may cause irritability; takes longer than with other medications to see clinical changes

TABLE 17–5. Bipolar and psychotic disorders: evidence-based medications *(continued)*

Medication name	Half-life (hours)	Usual teenage starting dosage (mg)	FDA maximum daily doses (mg; approval ages)	Available doses (mg)	Conditions with RCT support	Editorial comments
Quetiapine (Seroquel)	7	25 bid	800 (≥13 schizophrenia, ≥10 bipolar mania)	25, 50, 100, 200, 300, 400 tablets	Schizophrenia, bipolar mania	Pills are larger and so might be harder to swallow; noted anxiolytic properties
Ziprasidone (Geodon)	7	10 qam	160 in adults (not approved for children)	20, 40, 60, 80 capsules	Schizophrenia, bipolar mania	Greater risk of QT lengthening, so electrocardiogram monitoring is necessary; not a first-line option for children

TABLE 17–5. Bipolar and psychotic disorders: evidence-based medications *(continued)*

Medication name	Half-life (hours)	Usual teenage starting dosage (mg)	FDA maximum daily doses (mg; approval ages)	Available doses (mg)	Conditions with RCT support	Editorial comments
Olanzapine (Zyprexa)	30	2.5 qam	20 (≥13 schizophrenia, ≥13 bipolar mania, ≥10 bipolar depression, with fluoxetine)	2.5, 5, 7.5, 10, 15, 20 tablets	Schizophrenia, bipolar mania, bipolar depression	Has rapid benefits but greatest risk of weight gain and lipid changes in this group
Paliperidone (Invega)	23	3 qd	12 (≥12 schizophrenia)	1.5, 3, 6, 9 tablets	Schizophrenia	Major active metabolite of risperidone; similar risk of hyperprolactinemia

TABLE 17–5. Bipolar and psychotic disorders: evidence-based medications *(continued)*

Medication name	Half-life (hours)	Usual teenage starting dosage (mg)	FDA maximum daily doses (mg; approval ages)	Available doses (mg)	Conditions with RCT support	Editorial comments
Lurasidone	18	20 qd	80 (10–17 bipolar depression, 13–17 schizophrenia)	20, 40, 60, 80 tablets	Schizophrenia, bipolar depression	Take with food, weight neutral in kids
Asenapine	24	2.5 SL bid	20 (10–17 bipolar mania)	2.5, 5, 10 sublingual	Bipolar mania	Sublingual dissolve, oral paresthesia seen more often in kids

Note. RCT=randomized controlled trial; SL=sublingual.

azine (≥1 year old) for severe aggression, and thioridazine (≥2 years old) for schizophrenia. However, concern about adverse effects, chiefly movement disorders, limits contemporary use of these medications in children and adolescents.

Monitoring for Adverse Effects

When we prescribe a medication to a child or an adolescent, we take responsibility for monitoring for the development of known adverse effects. The tables in the following subsections are drawn from the published literature (Hilt 2012) and from adverse effect labeling from medication manufacturers (U.S. Food and Drug Administration 1999).

Stimulants

Stimulants (e.g., methylphenidate, dextroamphetamine) are usually well tolerated, but they often cause decreased appetite and insomnia (Table 17–6). Making adjustments to the dose and duration of action typically mitigates these problems. Tracking growth on a growth curve greatly helps with recognizing problems with weight gain (Table 17–7). With long-term use, there could be a decrease of 1–2 cm in final predicted adult height (Wolraich et al. 2019). Sometimes stimulants cause irritability or dysphoria, which may resolve if the patient switches to the other family of stimulant. Excessive doses can cause cognitive dulling. Stimulants often cause a very slight elevation in heart rate or blood pressure that is almost always clinically insignificant, but we screen for outlier responses via a vital signs check after initiation. A tic disorder is not really considered a contraindication for stimulant use because tics are just as likely to increase or decrease temporarily during stimulant use (Pringsheim and Steeves 2011).

Selective Serotonin Reuptake Inhibitors

Common side effects associated with SSRIs include a change in appetite that can lead to weight gain or loss and a sleep change that may include dreams becoming more vivid (Table 17–8). Diminished sex drive is common, although this problem is less notable for adolescents than for adults. Because platelets use serotonin for aggregation signaling, easier

TABLE 17–6. Highlights of adverse effects of stimulants

Common

    Decreased appetite

    Nausea

    Weight loss

    Insomnia

    Headaches

    Stomachaches

    Dry mouth

Less common

    Irritability

    Dysphoria

    Cognitive dulling

    Obsessiveness

    Anxiety

    Tics

    Dizziness

    Blood pressure and pulse rate elevation

Notable rare reactions

    Seizure

    Hallucinations

    Mania

    Loss of adult height potential

bruising may occur. Taking very high SSRI doses or combining serotonin agents could result in serotonin syndrome, which includes agitation, ataxia, diarrhea, hyperreflexia, mental status changes, tremor, and hyperthermia. Manic symptoms occur rarely as a side effect of SSRIs; their occurrence is not proof that the child will develop bipolar disorder. SSRIs have a common risk of causing irritability or agitation,

TABLE 17–7. Suggestions for monitoring of stimulants

Record height and weight growth curve at baseline and at each follow-up, at least every 6 months.

Measure blood pressure and pulse rate at baseline and after initiation of medication.

Monitor refill dates to identify signs of medication diversion.

Readminister ADHD symptom rating scale until remission is achieved.

which, if added to significant anxiety or depression, is one possible reason why there is a reported twofold increase in self-harm thoughts early in treatment when youth use SSRIs versus a placebo. Clinicians should discuss this FDA black box suicidality warning with patients and caregivers when prescribing an SSRI, along with the need for early treatment monitoring. Safe SSRI use involves examining a patient for adverse effects at around 2 weeks and again at 4–6 weeks after initiation to screen for worsening mood or irritability (Table 17–9) (Bridge et al. 2007).

Newer-Generation Antipsychotics

Antipsychotics for children and adolescents are typically initiated by mental health specialists, but primary care clinicians often find themselves in the role of providing refills or monitoring. Patients can experience significant adverse effects from these medications (Table 17–10). Weight gain is the most common problem, with patients in some trials gaining an average of more than 10 pounds in just 3 months of medication use (Correll et al. 2009). Weight gain seems to occur more frequently in children than in adults—for instance, aripiprazole and risperidone have been found to cause equal degrees of weight gain in children, a finding that contradicts the adult literature (Correll et al. 2009). Muscle stiffness or dystonia may occur, particularly during initial use. Clinicians can warn a family to keep over-the-counter diphenhydramine around as an available antidote. Sedation is common while taking antipsychotics, but this might be managed through bedtime dosing. A metabolic syndrome of elevated levels of blood glucose, cholesterol, and triglycerides may oc-

TABLE 17–8. Highlights of adverse effects of selective serotonin reuptake inhibitors

Common

Insomnia

Sedation

Appetite increase

Appetite decrease

Nausea

Dry mouth

Headache

Sexual dysfunction

Less common

Agitation

Restlessness

Impulsivity

Irritability

Silliness

Dizziness

Tremor

Constipation

Diarrhea

Notable rare reactions

Suicidal thoughts

Serotonin syndrome

Easy bleeding

Hyponatremia

Mania

Prolonged QT interval

TABLE 17–9. Suggestions for monitoring of selective serotonin reuptake inhibitors

Record height and weight at baseline and at each follow-up, at least every 6 months.

Inquire about increased irritability or agitation at 2 weeks and at 4–6 weeks after initiation.

Inquire about new or worsened suicidal thoughts at 2 weeks and at 4–6 weeks after initiation.

Inquire about new bleeding or bruising at least once after initiation.

Repeat disorder-specific rating scale(s) until remission is achieved. It takes 4–6 weeks to see benefits from a given dose.

cur for which regular blood tests are needed. A physical sense of restlessness (akathisia) or agitation may occur without parents realizing that this can be a side effect. The opposite could occur as well: medication-induced parkinsonism could decrease movement. One of the most worrisome side effects that we watch for is neuroleptic malignant syndrome, a severe febrile, systemic allergic reaction that typically occurs in the first few months of use (Neuhut et al. 2009). Families also must be warned about a small, but cumulative and dose-related, risk of tardive dyskinesia, which is a potentially permanent repetitive involuntary movement disorder caused by antipsychotics. Although similarly rare, the possibility of neuroleptic malignant syndrome and tardive dyskinesia needs to be part of the ongoing risk-benefit analysis around the use of these medications. Monitoring for tardive dyskinesia (Table 17–11) usually involves biannual examinations with the Abnormal Involuntary Movement Scale (AIMS) for any new-onset abnormal involuntary movements (McClellan et al. 2013).

Recording Adverse Medication Effects

If a child or an adolescent experiences an adverse effect of a medication prescribed for the treatment of a mental disorder, DSM-5-TR provides direction on how to record this information in the medical record (American Psychiatric Association 2022, pp. 807–819). We include Table 17–12 as a shorthand list

TABLE 17–10. Highlights of adverse effects of newer-generation antipsychotics

Common

Weight gain

Muscle rigidity

Parkinsonism

Constipation

Dry mouth

Dizziness

Somnolence or fatigue

Less common

Tremors

Nausea or abdominal pain

Akathisia (restlessness)

Headache

Agitation

Orthostasis

Elevated glucose level

Elevated levels of cholesterol and triglycerides

Notable rare reactions

Tardive dyskinesia

Neuroleptic malignant syndrome

Lowered blood cell counts

Elevated liver enzymes

Prolonged QT interval

Tachycardia

for recording a movement disorder or other adverse medication effect that is a focus of clinical attention or that may otherwise affect the diagnosis, course, prognosis, or treatment of a patient's mental disorder. A condition listed in the table

TABLE 17–11. Suggestions for monitoring of newer-generation antipsychotics

Record height and weight growth curve at baseline and at each follow-up, at least every 6 months.

Measure blood pressure and pulse rate at baseline and after initiation of medication.

Monitor levels of fasting blood glucose, triglycerides, and cholesterol every 6 months.

Obtain a complete blood cell count with differential once after initiation.

Inform the family about home monitoring for neuroleptic malignant syndrome and tardive dyskinesia.

Administer the Abnormal Involuntary Movement Scale (AIMS) every 6 months.

Adjust medication until remission is achieved.

Repeat the risk-benefit analysis every 6 months to wean the patient off the medication when appropriate.

may be coded if it is a reason for the current visit or helps to explain the need for a test, procedure, or treatment. Conditions and problems from this list also may be included in the medical record as useful information on circumstances that may affect the patient's care, regardless of their relevance to the current visit.

TABLE 17–12. ICD-10-CM codes for adverse medication effects

ICD-10-CM code	Disorder, condition, or problem
G21.11	Antipsychotic medication–and other dopamine receptor blocking agent–induced parkinsonism
G21.19	Other medication-induced parkinsonism
G21.0	Neuroleptic malignant syndrome
G24.02	Medication-induced acute dystonia
G25.71	Medication-induced acute akathisia
G24.01	Tardive dyskinesia
G24.09	Tardive dystonia
G25.71	Tardive akathisia
G25.1	Medication-induced postural tremor
G25.79	Other medication-induced movement disorder
T43.205A	Antidepressant discontinuation syndrome, initial encounter
T43.205D	Antidepressant discontinuation syndrome, subsequent encounter
T43.205S	Antidepressant discontinuation syndrome, sequelae
T50.905A	Other adverse effect of medication, initial encounter
T50.905D	Other adverse effect of medication, subsequent encounter
T50.905S	Other adverse effect of medication, sequelae

Source. World Health Organization 1992.

Chapter 18

Advancing Mental Health Care for Young People Through Practice, Education, Research, and Advocacy

Every day, we hear about a child or an adolescent who needs mental health care but cannot secure the care they need. Every day, we meet an adult whose mental distress and illness went unrecognized and unaddressed in their own formative years. We see that the needs for mental health services for children and adolescents are unmet.

As academic psychiatrists, we are grateful for our opportunities to care for patients as clinicians, to teach students and trainees to someday replace us as clinicians, and to conduct research that informs the clinical practice of other clinicians. However, we cannot accept every opportunity for clinical care, teaching, and research that is presented.

We cannot even accept the ideas that simply occur to us. Like many academics, we keep lists of ideas we hope to get to but realize that we would be fortunate to be able to address fewer than half of them. To end this book, we offer a decidedly incomplete list of ideas for practice, education, and research. We offer this incomplete conclusion both as a reminder that the work of caring for children and adolescents in mental distress is incomplete and as an invitation to join us in improving the lives of young people with mental illness. Select an idea, read the available literature on the idea, find academic or community partners to help you, and then begin.

Practice

1. Recognize and reduce adverse childhood experiences.
2. Minimize inappropriate use of antipsychotics, espe-

cially antipsychotic polypharmacy, among children and adolescents without psychotic disorders.

3. Develop outcome-based and quality improvement measures that are aligned with the goals of patients and caregivers rather than those of third-party payers and regulators.

4. Reduce the use of seclusion and restraint in pediatric psychiatric hospitals.

5. Increase the adoption rate for children in long-term foster care.

6. Improve trauma support services for children and families experiencing foster care.

7. Use social media peer networks to deliver some forms of mental health services.

8. Increase the use of specific DSM-5-TR (American Psychiatric Association 2022) diagnoses, as opposed to unspecified and otherwise specified diagnoses, in community settings.

9. Decrease stigma, both public and professional, around mental illness and mental health care.

10. Increase access to evidence-based behavioral- and psychological-based treatments for mental illness in children and adolescents.

11. Increase success rates for mental health service referrals through addressing access barriers.

12. Develop crisis support services that would effectively diminish the use of emergency rooms for child mental health.

13. Develop dashboards that chart progress toward health equity in clinical outcomes.

Education

1. Integrate community-based mental health care into nonspecialty settings.

2. Innovate curriculum to more effectively teach mental health diagnosis and treatment to nonspecialty clinicians.

3. Teach culturally informed care that considers a young person's ethnicity, language, faith, sexuality, and gender orientation.

4. Develop strategies to provide high-quality early childhood education to all children.

5. Teach individual caregivers ways to maintain and strengthen the resiliency of children.
6. Incorporate mental health training into the training of coaches, teachers, and other adults in caring professions.
7. Increase understanding of the effects of adverse childhood experiences and reduce their incidence.
8. Teach parents and caregivers the benefits of predictable habits at home and school for a child's development.
9. Help educators understand and implement effective strategies to prevent and reduce bullying.
10. Use public health strategies to promote greater use of effective parenting practices.
11. Develop local behavioral health systems that support schools' multitiered systems of support.
12. Help schools develop strategies for safe, in-person education.

Research

1. Improve the reliability of the disruptive mood dysregulation disorder diagnosis and evaluate its best treatment in children and adolescents.
2. Study cannabis and its association with psychotic changes in adolescents, identifying harm reduction strategies.
3. Evaluate the childhood risk rate of tardive dyskinesia from newer-generation antipsychotics.
4. Comparatively study interventions for child mental health conditions—for example, what is the most effective treatment for pediatric bipolar disorder?
5. Study long-term outcomes (including undesired effects) from the use of psychotropic medications in children.
6. Test the effectiveness in children of antidepressants released over the past decade.
7. Study α_2-agonists and selective serotonin reuptake inhibitors for their degree of benefit for treating childhood PTSD symptoms.
8. Study the potential benefits of computer-delivered (i.e., via video game, texting, and social media formats) psychosocial interventions on child mental health symptoms.
9. Study psychotherapeutic interventions (such as dialectical behavior therapy) specifically for their ability to reduce the risk of suicide among high-risk adolescents.

10. Study psychosocial and behavioral interventions for autism spectrum disorders that may be more practical to implement than full-time applied behavior analysis therapy.
11. Study the differential experiences of patients and clinicians treated through telepsychiatry.

Integration of Care

Finally, there is a growing recognition that integrating mental and physical health services for young people improves the experience of care and treatment outcomes while (potentially) reducing the total cost of care. The jury is still out on that last point, but it has become accepted that better integration of care can make it easier for families to access services and can yield improved treatment outcomes. What remains undetermined is how this integration of care should be designed or how it would work in child mental health. Over the next decade, we hope to witness and participate in major improvements in integrated care systems.

As you see children and adolescents for care, consider whether the system in which you are seeing them could be transformed into an effective integrated care system for children and adolescents. By referencing what has been learned about effective integrated care systems in adults, and adding to that our own integrated care experiences and the views of the American Academy of Child and Adolescent Psychiatry, we have created a list of what an integrated care system should include to function well for both providers and families, as summarized in Table 18–1.

TABLE 18–1. Elements of an effective integrated mental health care system for young people

1. Screening for early detection of behavioral health problems

2. Co-location of mental health services without visual service separation for families

3. Licensed mental health clinician(s) present on site

4. Care manager/care coordinator(s) facilitating regular primary care and mental health clinician communication

5. Primary care clinicians can rapidly access child and adolescent psychiatric consultations

6. Evidence-based workflows and care pathways are operationalized for common conditions

7. Health care records integrate physical and mental health care

8. Training, regular case supervision and support are provided for clinic staff

9. Active monitoring of patient care, via rating scales or verbal check-ins, affect treatment plans which pursue measurable treatment goal

10. Reimbursement sustains the care system

Source. American Academy of Child and Adolescent Psychiatry 2012; Isaacs and Mitchell 2024.

References

Achenbach TM: Manual for the Child Behavior Checklist/4–18 and 1991 Profile. Burlington, VT, Department of Psychiatry, University of Vermont, 1991

Achenbach TM: Manual for the Child Behavior Checklist/2–3 and 1992 Profile. Burlington, VT, Department of Psychiatry, University of Vermont, 1992

Aggarwal NK, Lam P, Jiménez-Solomon O, et al: An online training module on the Cultural Formulation Interview: the case of New York State. Psychiatr Serv 69(11):1135–1137, 2018 30041589

Alarcón RD, Frank JB: The Psychotherapy of Hope: The Legacy of Persuasion and Healing. Baltimore, MD, Johns Hopkins University Press, 2011

Allcott H, Braghieri L, Eichmeyer S, et al: The welfare effects of social media. Am Econ Rev 110(3):629–676, 2020

American Academy of Child and Adolescent Psychiatry: Best principles for integration of child psychiatry into the pediatric health home. June 2012. Available at: www.aacap.org/App_Themes/AACAP/docs/clinical_practice_center/systems_of_care/best_principles_for_integration_of_child_psychiatry_into_the_pediatric_health_home_2012.pdf. Accessed August 31, 2015.

American Psychiatric Association: Diagnostic and Statistical Manual of Mental Disorders, 3rd Edition. Washington, DC, American Psychiatric Association, 1980

American Psychiatric Association: Diagnostic and Statistical Manual of Mental Disorders, 4th Edition. Washington, DC, American Psychiatric Association, 1994

American Psychiatric Association: Diagnostic and Statistical Manual of Mental Disorders, 5th Edition. Arlington, VA, American Psychiatric Association, 2013

American Psychiatric Association: Diagnostic and Statistical Manual of Mental Disorders, 5th Edition, Text Revision. Washington, DC, American Psychiatric Association, 2022

Bäärnhielm S, Scarpinati Rosso M: The Cultural Formulation: a model to combine nosology and patients' life context in psychiatric diagnostic practice. Transcult Psychiatry 46(3):406–428, 2009 19837779

Beloglovsky M, Daly L: Early Learning Theories Made Visible. St. Paul, MN, Redleaf, 2015

Berganza CE, Mezzich JE: Guía Latinoamericana de Diagnóstico Psiquiátrico. Guadalajara, Jalisco, México, 2004

Birmaher B, Brent D, Bernet W, et al: Practice parameter for the assessment and treatment of children and adolescents with depressive disorders. J Am Acad Child Adolesc Psychiatry 46(11):1503–1526, 2007 18049300

Birmaher B, Gill MK, Axelson DA, et al: Longitudinal trajectories and associated baseline predictors in youths with bipolar spectrum disorders. Am J Psychiatry 171(9):990–999, 2014 24874203

Bitsko RH, Claussen AH, Lichstein J, et al: Mental health surveillance among children—United States, 2013–2019. MMWR Suppl 71(2)(Suppl-2):1–42, 2022 35202359

Braüner JV, Johansen LM, Roesbjerg T, et al: Off-label prescription of psychopharmacological drugs in child and adolescent psychiatry. J Clin Psychopharmacol 36(5):500–507, 2016 27529772

Bridge JA, Iyengar S, Salary CB, et al: Clinical response and risk for reported suicidal ideation and suicide attempts in pediatric antidepressant treatment: a meta-analysis of randomized controlled trials. JAMA 297(15):1683–1696, 2007 17440145

Buu A, Dipiazza C, Wang J, et al: Parent, family, and neighborhood effects on the development of child substance use and other psychopathology from preschool to the start of adulthood. J Stud Alcohol Drugs 70(4):489–498, 2009 19515288

Buxton D, Potter MP, Bostic JQ: Coping strategies for child bully-victims. Pediatr Ann 42(4):57–61, 2013 23556519

Cepeda C, Gotanco L: Psychiatric Interview of Children and Adolescents. Arlington, VA, American Psychiatric Association, 2017

Chen YF: Chinese Classification of Mental Disorders (CCMD-3): towards integration in international classification. Psychopathology 35(2-3):171–175, 2002 12145505

Chisolm MS, Lyketsos CG: Systematic Psychiatric Evaluation: A Step-by-Step Guide to Applying the Perspectives of Psychiatry. Baltimore, MD, Johns Hopkins University Press, 2012

Chorpita BF, Daleiden EL: Mapping evidence-based treatments for children and adolescents: application of the distillation and matching model to 615 treatments from 322 randomized trials. J Consult Clin Psychol 77(3):566–579, 2009 19485596

Christophersen ER, VanScoyoc SW: Treatments That Work With Children: Empirically Supported Strategies for Managing Childhood Problems, 2nd Edition. Washington, DC, American Psychological Association, 2013

Clark LA, Cuthbert B, Lewis-Fernández R, et al: Three approaches to understanding and classifying mental disorder: ICD-11, DSM-5, and the National Institute of Mental Health's research domain criteria (RDoC). Psychol Sci Public Interest 18(2):72–145, 2017 29211974

Cohen H: The nature, methods and purpose of diagnosis. Lancet 24(6227):23–25, 1943

Correll CU, Manu P, Olshanskiy V, et al: Cardiometabolic risk of second-generation antipsychotic medications during first-time use in children and adolescents. JAMA 302(16):1765–1773, 2009 19861668

Davanzo R, Copertino M, De Cunto A, et al: Antidepressant drugs and breastfeeding: a review of the literature. Breastfeed Med 6(2):89–98, 2011 20958101

Davis DE, Choe E, Meyers J, et al: Thankful for the little things: a meta-analysis of gratitude interventions. J Couns Psychol 63(1):20–31, 2016 26575348

de Haan AM, Boon AE, de Jong JT, et al: A meta-analytic review on treatment dropout in child and adolescent outpatient mental health care. Clin Psychol Rev 33(5):698–711, 2013 23742782

DelRosso LM, Picchietti DL, Spruyt K, et al: Restless sleep in children: a systematic review. Sleep Med Rev 56:101406, 2021 33341437

Díaz E, Añez LM, Silva M, et al: Using the Cultural Formulation Interview to build culturally sensitive services. Psychiatr Serv 68(2):112–114, 2017 27799018

Dickson SJ, Kuhnert RL, Lavell CH, et al: Impact of psychotherapy for children and adolescents with anxiety disorders on global and domain-specific functioning: a systematic review and meta-analysis. Clin Child Fam Psychol Rev 25(4):720–736, 2022 35794304

Digman JM: Personality structure: emergence of the five-factor model. Annu Rev Psychol 41:417–440, 1990

Dulcan MK (ed): Dulcan's Textbook of Child and Adolescent Psychiatry, 3rd Edition. Washington, DC, American Psychiatric Association Publishing, 2022

Dvir Y, Ford JD, Hill M, et al: Childhood maltreatment, emotional dysregulation, and psychiatric comorbidities. Harv Rev Psychiatry 22(3):149–161, 2014 24704784

Eaton DK, Kann L, Kinchen S, et al: Youth risk behavior surveillance—United States, 2007. MMWR Surveill Summ 57(4):1–131, 2008 18528314

Egger HL, Emde RN: Developmentally sensitive diagnostic criteria for mental health disorders in early childhood: the Diagnostic and Statistical Manual of Mental Disorders-IV, the Research Diagnostic Criteria-Preschool Age, and the Diagnostic Classification of Mental Health and Developmental Disorders of Infancy and Early Childhood-Revised. Am Psychol 66(2):95–106, 2011 21142337

Emanuel EJ, Emanuel LL: Four models of the physician-patient relationship. JAMA 267(16):2221–2226, 1992 1556799

Emmons RA, McCullough ME: Counting blessings versus burdens: an experimental investigation of gratitude and subjective well-being in daily life. J Pers Soc Psychol 84(2):377–389, 2003 12585811

Emslie GJ, Mayes T, Porta G, et al: Treatment of Resistant Depression in Adolescents (TORDIA): week 24 outcomes. Am J Psychiatry 167(7):782–791, 2010 20478877

Estroff SE, Henderson GE: Social and cultural contributions to health, difference, and inequality, in The Social Medicine Reader, 2nd Edition, Vol 2. Edited by Henderson G, Estroff SE. Durham, NC, Duke University Press, 2005, pp 4–26

Feinstein AR: Clinical Judgment. Baltimore, MD, Williams & Wilkins, 1967

First MB: DSM-5-TR Handbook of Differential Diagnosis. Washington, DC, American Psychiatric Publishing, 2022

Folstein MF, Folstein SE, McHugh PR: "Mini-mental state": a practical method for grading the cognitive state of patients for the clinician. J Psychiatr Res 12(3):189–198, 1975 1202204

Ford CA, Millstein SG, Halpern-Felsher BL, et al: Influence of physician confidentiality assurances on adolescents' willingness to disclose information and seek future health care: a randomized controlled trial. JAMA 278(12):1029–1034, 1997 9307357

Fornaro M, Maritan E, Ferranti R, et al: Lithium exposure during pregnancy and the postpartum period: a systematic review and meta-analysis of safety and efficacy outcomes. Am J Psychiatry 177(1):76–92, 2020 31623458

Gerber RJ, Wilks T, Erdie-Lalena C: Developmental milestones: motor development. Pediatr Rev 31(7):267–276, quiz 277, 2010 20595440

Gerber RJ, Wilks T, Erdie-Lalena C: Developmental milestones 3: social-emotional development. Pediatr Rev 32(12):533–536, 2011 22135423

Girand HL, Litkowiec S, Sohn M: Attention-deficit/hyperactivity disorder and psychotropic polypharmacy prescribing trends. Pediatrics 146(1):e20192832, 2020 32487590

Gold MA, Seningen AE: Interviewing adolescents, in American Academy of Pediatrics Textbook of Pediatric Care. Edited by McInerny TK. Washington, DC, American Academy of Pediatrics, 2009, pp 1331–1337

Hanington L, Ramchandani P, Stein A: Parental depression and child temperament: assessing child to parent effects in a longitudinal population study. Infant Behav Dev 33(1):88–95, 2010 20056283

Hanley GP, Iwata BA, McCord BE: Functional analysis of problem behavior: a review. J Appl Behav Anal 36(2):147–185, 2003 12858983

Hazell P, Mirzaie M: Tricyclic drugs for depression in children and adolescents. Cochrane Database Syst Rev 2013(6):CD002317, 2013 23780719

Hilt RJ: Monitoring psychiatric medications in children. Pediatr Ann 41(4):157–163, 2012 22494208

Hilt RJ: Primary care principles for child mental health, version 121. 2024. Available at: www.seattlechildrens.org/healthcare-professionals/community-providers/pal/resources. Accessed June 6, 2024.

Hughes K, Bellis MA, Hardcastle KA, et al: The effect of multiple adverse childhood experiences on health: a systematic review and meta-analysis. Lancet Public Health 2(8):e356–e366, 2017 29253477

Hunt MG, Marx R, Lipson C, et al: No more FOMO: limiting social media decreases loneliness and depression. J Soc Clin Psychol 37(10):751–768, 2018

Insel TR, Quirion R: Psychiatry as a clinical neuroscience discipline. JAMA 294(17):2221–2224, 2005 16264165

Insel T, Cuthbert B, Garvey M, et al: Research domain criteria (RDoC): toward a new classification framework for research on mental disorders. Am J Psychiatry 167(7):748–751, 2010 20595427

Isaacs AN, Mitchell EKL: Mental health integrated care models in primary care and factors that contribute to their effective implementation: a scoping review. In J Ment Health Syst 18(1):5, 2024 38331913

Ivey-Stephenson AZ, Demissie Z, Crosby AE, et al: Suicidal ideation and behaviors among high school students—Youth Risk Behavior Survey, United States, 2020. MMWR Suppl 69(Suppl 1):47–55, 2020 32817610

Jarvis GE, Kirmayer LJ, Gómez-Carrillo A, et al: Update on the Cultural Formulation Interview. Focus Am Psychiatr Publ 18(1):40–46, 2020 32047396

Jellinek M, Patel BP, Froehle MC (eds): Bright Futures in Practice: Mental Health, Vol. 1: Practice Guide. Arlington, VA, National Center for Education in Maternal and Child Health, 2002. Available at: www.brightfutures.org/mentalhealth. Accessed August 31, 2015.

Johnstone L, Boyle M, Cromby J, et al: The Power Threat Meaning Framework: Towards the Identification of Patterns in Emotional Distress, Unusual Experiences and Troubled or Troubling Behaviour as an Alternative to Functional Psychiatric Diagnosis. Leicester, UK, British Psychological Society, 2018

Jonas BS, Gu Q, Albertorio-Diaz JR: Psychotropic Medication Use Among Adolescents: United States, 2005–2010 (NCHS Data Brief No 135). Hyattsville, MD, National Center for Health Statistics, 2013

Kendall PC: Child and Adolescent Therapy: Cognitive-Behavioral Procedures, 4th Edition. New York, Guilford, 2012

Kendell R, Jablensky A: Distinguishing between the validity and utility of psychiatric diagnoses. Am J Psychiatry 160(1):4–12, 2003 12505793

Kendler KS: The dappled nature of causes of psychiatric illness: replacing the organic-functional/hardware-software dichotomy with empirically based pluralism. Mol Psychiatry 17(4):377–388, 2012 22230881

Keshavarzi H, Khan F, Alu B, et al: Applying Islamic Principles to Clinical Mental Health Care. New York, Routledge, 2020

Kessler RC, Chiu WT, Demler O, et al: Prevalence, severity, and comorbidity of 12-month DSM-IV disorders in the National Comorbidity Survey Replication. Arch Gen Psychiatry 62(6):617–627, 2005 15939839(erratum Arch Gen Psychiatry 62:709, 2005)

Kinghorn WA: Whose disorder? A constructive MacIntyrean critique of psychiatric nosology. J Med Philos 36(2):187–205, 2011 21357652

Knight JR, Sherritt L, Shrier LA, et al: Validity of the CRAFFT substance abuse screening test among adolescent clinic patients. Arch Pediatr Adolesc Med 156(6):607–614, 2002 12038895

Kotov R, Krueger RF, Watson D, et al: The Hierarchical Taxonomy of Psychopathology (HiTOP): a dimensional alternative to traditional nosologies. J Abnorm Psychol 126(4):454–477, 2017 28333488

Kovess-Masfety V, Van Engelen J, Stone L, et al: Unmet need for specialty mental health services among children across Europe. Psychiatr Serv 68(8):789–795, 2017 28366116

Kozak MJ, Cuthbert BN: The NIMH Research Domain Criteria Initiative: background, issues, and pragmatics. Psychophysiology 53(3):286–297, 2016 26877115

Lanza di Scalea T, Wisner KL: Antidepressant medication use during breastfeeding. Clin Obstet Gynecol 52(3):483–497, 2009 19661763

Lavigne JV, Lebailly SA, Gouze KR, et al: Treating oppositional defiant disorder in primary care: a comparison of three models. J Pediatr Psychol 33(5):449–461, 2008 17956932

Lewis-Fernández R, Aggarwal NK, Hinton L, et al: DSM-5 Handbook on the Cultural Formulation Interview. Washington, DC, American Psychiatric Publishing, 2016

Lim R: Clinical Manual of Cultural Psychiatry, 2nd Edition. Arlington, VA, American Psychiatric Association, 2015

Lizardi D, Oquendo MA, Graver R: Clinical pitfalls in the diagnosis of ataque de nervios: a case study. Transcult Psychiatry 46(3):463–486, 2009 19837782

Loy JH, Merry SN, Hetrick SE, et al: Atypical antipsychotics for disruptive behaviour disorders in children and youths. Cochrane Database Syst Rev 8(8):CD008559, 2017 28791693

MacIntyre AC: Dependent Rational Animals: Why Human Beings Need the Virtues. Chicago, IL, Open Court Publishing, 2012

Maza MT, Fox KA, Kwon SJ, et al: Association of habitual checking behaviors on social media with longitudinal functional brain development. JAMA Pediatr 177(2):160–167, 2023 36595277

McCartney K, Philips DA: Blackwell Handbook of Early Childhood Development. Malden, MA, Blackwell, 2006

McClellan J, Stock S; American Academy of Child and Adolescent Psychiatry (AACAP) Committee on Quality Issues (CQI): Practice parameter for the assessment and treatment of children and adolescents with schizophrenia. J Am Acad Child Adolesc Psychiatry 52(9):976–990, 2013 23972700

McLaughlin MR: Speech and language delay in children. Am Fam Physician 83(10):1183–1188, 2011 21568252

McVoy M, Findling RL (eds): Clinical Manual of Child and Adolescent Psychopharmacology, 2nd Edition. Washington, DC, American Psychiatric Publishing, 2013

McVoy M, Findling RL (eds): Clinical Manual of Child and Adolescent Psychopharmacology, 3rd Edition. Arlington, VA, American Psychiatric Association Publishing, 2017

Meltzer LJ, Johnson C, Crosette J, et al: Prevalence of diagnosed sleep disorders in pediatric primary care practices. Pediatrics 125(6):e1410–e1418, 2010 20457689

Meltzer-Brody S, Colquhoun H, Riesenberg R, et al: Brexanolone injection in post-partum depression: two multicentre, double-blind, randomised, placebo-controlled, phase 3 trials. Lancet 392(10152):1058–1070, 2018 30177236

Merikangas KR, He JP, Burstein M, et al: Lifetime prevalence of mental disorders in U.S. adolescents: results from the National Comorbidity Survey Replication—Adolescent Supplement (NCS-A). J Am Acad Child Adolesc Psychiatry 49(10):980–989, 2010 20855043

Mills S, Wolitzky-Taylor K, Xiao AQ, et al: Training on the DSM-5 Cultural Formulation Interview improves cultural competence in general psychiatry residents: a multi-site study. Acad Psychiatry 40(5):829–834, 2016 27093964

Mindell J, Owens J: A Clinical Guide to Pediatric Sleep: Diagnosis and Management of Pediatric Sleep Problems, 2nd Edition. Philadelphia, PA, Lippincott, Williams & Wilkins, 2009

Mises R, Quemada N, Botbol M, et al: French classification for child and adolescent mental disorders. Psychopathology 35(2-3):176–180, 2002 12145506

Mohatt J, Bennett SM, Walkup JT: Treatment of separation, generalized, and social anxiety disorders in youths. Am J Psychiatry 171(7):741–748, 2014 24874020

Mooney CG: Theories of Childhood: An Introduction to Dewey, Montessori, Erikson, Piaget, and Vygotsky, 2nd Edition. St. Paul, MN, Redleaf Press, 2013

Morin JG, Afzali MH, Bourque J, et al: A population-based analysis of the relationship between substance use and adolescent cognitive development. Am J Psychiatry 176(2):98–106, 2019 30278790

Murphy SE, Capitão LP, Giles SLC, et al: The knowns and unknowns of SSRI treatment in young people with depression and anxiety: efficacy, predictors, and mechanisms of action. Lancet Psychiatry 8(9):824–835, 2021 34419187

Nakane Y, Nakane H: Classification systems for psychiatric diseases currently used in Japan. Psychopathology 35(2-3):191–194, 2002 12145509

National Institute of Mental Health: Ask Suicide-Screening Questions (ASQ) toolkit. Bethesda, MD, National Institute of Mental Health. 2024. Available at: www.nimh.nih.gov/research/research-conducted-at-nimh/asq-toolkit-materials. Accessed June 6, 2024.

Neuhut R, Lindenmayer J-P, Silva R: Neuroleptic malignant syndrome in children and adolescents on atypical antipsychotic medication: a review. J Child Adolesc Psychopharmacol 19(4):415–422, 2009 19702493

Nurcombe B: Diagnosis and treatment planning in child and adolescent mental health problems, in IACAPAP e-Textbook of Child and Adolescent Mental Health. Edited by Rey JM. Geneva, Switzerland, International Association for Child and Adolescent Psychiatry and Allied Professions, 2014, pp 1–21

Nussbaum AM: The Pocket Guide to the DSM-5-TR® Diagnostic Exam. Washington, DC, American Psychiatric Association Publishing, 2022

Orben A, Przybylski AK, Blakemore SJ, et al: Windows of developmental sensitivity to social media. Nat Commun 13(1):1649, 2022 35347142

Otero-Ojeda AA: Third Cuban Glossary of Psychiatry (GC-3): key features and contributions. Psychopathology 35(2-3):181–184, 2002 12145507

Paschetta E, Berrisford G, Coccia F, et al: Perinatal psychiatric disorders: an overview. Am J Obstet Gynecol 210(6):501–509.e6, 2014 24113256

Pearlstein T: Use of psychotropic medication during pregnancy and the postpartum period. Womens Health (Lond Engl) 9(6):605–615, 2013 24161312

Pringsheim T, Steeves T: Pharmacological treatment for attention deficit hyperactivity disorder (ADHD) in children with comorbid tic disorders. Cochrane Database Syst Rev (4):CD007990, 2011 21491404

Pringsheim T, Stewart DG, Chan P, et al: The pharmacoepidemiology of psychotropic medication use in Canadian children from 2012 to 2016. J Child Adolesc Psychopharmacol 29(10):740–745, 2019 31355670

Radden J, Sadler JZ: The Virtuous Psychiatrist: Character Ethics in Psychiatric Practice. New York, Oxford University Press, 2010

Reynolds CR, Kamphaus RW: BASC: Behavior Assessment System for Children, 3rd Edition. Circle Pines, MN, American Guidance Service, 2015

Riehm KE, Feder KA, Tormohlen KN, et al: Associations between time spent using social media and internalizing and externalizing problems among US youth. JAMA Psychiatry 76(12):1266–1273, 2019 31509167

Romano E, Babchishin L, Marquis R, et al: Childhood maltreatment and educational outcomes. Trauma Violence Abuse 16(4):418–437, 2015 24920354

Roos J, Werbart A: Therapist and relationship factors influencing dropout from individual psychotherapy: a literature review. Psychother Res 23(4):394–418, 2013 23461273

Rushton J, Bruckman D, Kelleher K: Primary care referral of children with psychosocial problems. Arch Pediatr Adolesc Med 156(6):592–598, 2002 12038893

Satyanarayana VA, Lukose A, Srinivasan K: Maternal mental health in pregnancy and child behavior. Indian J Psychiatry 53(4):351–361, 2011 22303046

Schramm E, Klein DN, Elsaesser M, et al: Review of dysthymia and persistent depressive disorder: history, correlates, and clinical implications. Lancet Psychiatry 7(9):801–812, 2020 32828168

Scott BG, Sanders AFP, Graham RA, et al: Identity distress among youth exposed to natural disasters: associations with level of exposure, posttraumatic stress, and internalizing problems. Identity (Mahwah, NJ) 14(4):255–267, 2014 25505851

Shahrokh NC, Hales RE, Phillips KA, et al: The Language of Mental Health: A Glossary of Psychiatric Terms. Washington, DC, American Psychiatric Publishing, 2011

Silber TJ: Somatization disorders: diagnosis, treatment, and prognosis. Pediatr Rev 32(2):56–63, quiz 63–64, 2011 21285301

Substance Abuse and Mental Health Services Administration: Key substance use and mental health indicators in the United States: Results from the 2021 National Survey on Drug Use and Health (DHHS Publ No PEP22-07-01-005, NSDUH Series H-57). Rockville, MD, Substance Abuse and Mental Health Services Administration. 2022. Available at: www.samhsa.gov/data/sites/default/files/reports/rpt39443/2021NSDUHFFRRev010323.pdf. Accessed January 16, 2024.

Summers RF, Barber JP: Therapeutic alliance as a measurable psychotherapy skill. Acad Psychiatry 27(3):160–165, 2003 12969839

Task Force on Research Diagnostic Criteria: Infancy Preschool: Research diagnostic criteria for infants and preschool children: the process and empirical support. J Am Acad Child Adolesc Psychiatry 42(12):1504–1512, 2003 14627886

Tolliver DG, Lee LK, Patterson EE, et al: Disparities in school referrals for agitation and aggression to the emergency department. Acad Pediatr 22(4):598–605, 2022 34780998

U.S. Food and Drug Administration: Online label repository, 1999. Available at: http://labels.fda.gov. Accessed March 1, 2015.

U.S. Public Health Service: Mental Health: A Report of the Surgeon General. Rockville, MD, U.S. Public Health Service, 1999

VanderWeele TJ: Activities for flourishing: an evidence-based guide. J Posit Psychol Wellbeing 4(1):79–91, 2020

van Nierop M, Janssens M, Bruggeman R, et al: Evidence that transition from health to psychotic disorder can be traced to semi-ubiquitous environmental effects operating against background genetic risk. PLoS One 8(11):e76690, 2013 24223116

Vernon-Feagans L, Garrett-Peters P, Willoughby M, et al: Chaos, poverty, and parenting: predictors of early language development. Early Child Res Q 27(3):339–351, 2012 23049162

Weisz JR, Kazdin AE: Evidence-Based Psychotherapies for Children and Adolescents, 2nd Edition. New York, Guilford, 2010

Wilks T, Gerber RJ, Erdie-Lalena C: Developmental milestones: cognitive development. Pediatr Rev 31(9):364–367, 2010 20810700

Wolraich ML, Hagan JF Jr, Allan C, et al: Clinical Practice Guideline for the Diagnosis, Evaluation, and Treatment of Attention-Deficit/Hyperactivity Disorder in Children and Adolescents. Pediatrics 144(4):e20192528, 2019 31570648

World Health Organization: The ICD-10 Classification of Mental and Behavioural Disorders: Clinical Descriptions and Diagnostic Guidelines. Geneva, World Health Organization, 1992

Yackey K, Stukus K, Cohen D, et al: Off-label medication prescribing patterns in pediatrics: an update. Hosp Pediatr 9(3):186–193, 2019 30745323

Youngstrom EA, Prinstein MJ, Mash EJ, et al: Assessment of Disorders in Childhood and Adolescence, 5th Edition. New York, Guilford, 2022

Yuma-Guerrero PJ, Lawson KA, Velasquez MM, et al: Screening, brief intervention, and referral for alcohol use in adolescents: a systematic review. Pediatrics 130(1):115–122, 2012 22665407

Zero to Three: Diagnostic Classification of Mental Health and Developmental Disorders of Infancy and Early Childhood (DC: 0–5). Washington, DC, Zero to Three National Center, 2016

Index

Page numbers printed in **boldface** type refer to tables or figures.

Dextroamphetamine, **307, 311–313**

Diagnosis. *See also* Alternatives; Assessment; Differential diagnosis; DSM-5-TR; Exclusion criteria; Inclusion criteria; Misdiagnosis; Other specified diagnoses; Severity; Specifiers; Unspecified diagnoses; *specific disorders*

alternative systems of, 254, **255–257,** 258

categorical model of, 221

contents of current volume, 3–5

developmental stages and, 269

15-minute interview and, 69–79

multiaxial system of, 277–278

multistep approach to, 11–12

of neurodevelopmental disorders, 95–104

rating scales used in, 249–250, **251–253,** 254

30-minute interview and, 81–90

treatment plans and, 277–278

Diagnostic Classification of Mental Health and Development Disorders of Infancy and Early Childhood (DC:0-5), 260

Dialectical behavior therapy, **299**

Diarrhea, and opioid withdrawal, 172

Differential diagnosis
absence of mental disorder and, 211

of aggression, 26

comorbidity of mental disorders and, 210

conflict with caregiver and, 208–209

developmental stages or conflicts and, 208

intentional production of signs and symptoms, 207–208

medical conditions and, 209–210

substance use and, 209

Dimensional model, for diagnosis of personality disorders, 244–245

Diphenhydramine, 325

Disinhibited social engagement disorder, 130

Disorders, use of term, 278–279

Disorganized speech, and schizophrenia, 105

Disproportionate thoughts, and somatic symptom disorder, 133

Disruptive behavior, as common clinical concern, 38–42

Disruptive, impulse-control, and conduct disorders, DSM-5-TR and diagnosis of, 150–155, **204–205**

Disruptive mood dysregulation disorder
DSM-5-TR and diagnosis of, 116–117, **199**

irritable mood and, 46–47

Dissociation
amnesia and, 131

Guilt, and major depressive disorder, 113

Hallucinations
    alcohol withdrawal and, 159
    cannabis intoxication and, 163
    mental status examination and, 216
    schizophrenia and, 104–105, **197**
    sedative, hypnotic, or anxiolytic withdrawal and, 175
Hallucinogen(s). *See* Other hallucinogen use disorder
Hallucinogen persisting perception disorder, 165
Haloperidol, 305, 323
Hazardous situations. *See also* Safety
    alcohol use disorder and, 157
    cannabis use disorder and, 161
    inhalant use disorder and, 167
    opioid use disorder and, 170
    other (or unknown) substance use disorder and, 182–183
    phencyclidine use disorder and, 164–165
    sedative, hypnotic, or anxiolytic use disorder and, 173
    stimulant use disorder and, 176
    tobacco use disorder and, 180

Headache, and caffeine withdrawal, 160
Health care. *See also* Emergency departments; Hospitalization; Medical conditions; Primary care clinicians
    coding of problems with access in medical record, 192
    gender-affirming procedures or treatments, 149
    integration of mental health care with, 334, **335**
Hearing
    academic performance and, **33**
    developmental delay and, 37–38
Heart rate, and panic disorder, 119. *See also* Tachycardia
Hierarchical Taxonomy of Psychopathology (HiTOP), 258–259
Hoarding disorder, 124
Homelessness, coding of in medical record, 190
Home visit crisis services, 25
Hospitalization. *See also* Emergency departments
    postpartum maternal mental health and, 67
    suicidality and, 25, 58
Housing problems, coding of in medical record, 190
Humor, and establishment of therapeutic alliance, 7
Hydroxyzine, 56
Hyperactivity, and ADHD, 102–103, **196**

Hyperreactivity or hyporeactivity, and autism spectrum disorder, 99

Hypersomnia
major depressive disorder and, 113
stimulant withdrawal and, 179

Hypersomnolence disorder, 142–144

Hypervigilance, and PTSD, 127

Hypocretin deficiency, and narcolepsy, 144

Hypomania, and bipolar II disorder, **198**

Hypothyroidism, and withdrawn or sad mood, 42

ICD-10, and CM codes for adverse medication effects, **330.** *See also* World Health Organization

ICD-11, as alternative diagnostic system, 254, 258. *See also* World Health Organization; Z codes

Ideas of reference, and mental status examination, 216

Illness anxiety disorder, 134–135

Illusions, and mental status examination, 216

Impairment, and body-focused repetitive behaviors, 125

Impulsivity, and ADHD, 102–103, **196**

Inclusion criteria, for DSM-5-TR diagnoses
for alcohol use disorder, 156, 158–159
for anorexia nervosa, 136
for ADHD, 101–103

for autism spectrum disorder, 98–99
for bipolar I disorder, 108
for bipolar II disorder, 110–111
for body-focused repetitive behaviors, 124–125
for caffeine use disorder, 159–161
for cannabis use disorder, 161–163
for conduct disorder, 152–154
for depersonalization/derealization disorder, 131–132
for disruptive mood dysregulation disorder, 116–117
for dissociative amnesia, 131
for encopresis, 140
for enuresis, 139
for gambling disorder, 184–185
for gender dysphoria, 149
for generalized anxiety disorder, 121
for hypersomnolence disorder, 142–143
for illness anxiety disorder, 134–135
for inhalant use disorder, 167–169
for insomnia disorder, 141
for intellectual developmental disorder, 96
for intermittent explosive disorder, 151–152
for major depressive disorder, 113
for OCD, 122–124

Internet. *See* Social media; Web sites

Intoxication
  alcohol and, 158
  caffeine and, 159
  cannabis and, 162–163
  inhalants and, 168–169
  opioids and, 171
  other (or unknown) substance and, 183–184
  sedative, hypnotic, or anxiolytics and, 174–175
  stimulants and, 178

Intrusions, and PTSD, **201, 202**

IQ test scores, and academic performance, 34

Irritability
  caffeine withdrawal and, 160–161
  cannabis withdrawal and, 163
  as common concern, 45–47
  gambling disorder and, 184
  generalized anxiety disorder and, 121
  oppositional defiant disorder and, 150–151
  PTSD and, 127
  reactive attachment disorder and, 129
  screening questions for, 116
  SSRIs and, 45
  tobacco withdrawal and, 181

Judgment, and mental status examination, 217

Kendler, Kenneth, 207
Khyâl cap (wind attack), 122
Kleptomania, 155

Koro, 124

Labile mood, 45–47

Lacrimation, and opioid withdrawal, 172

Language. *See also* Screening; Speech
  aggression and limited skills in, 26
  gender-neutrality and, vii–viii
  psychiatric glossary in appendix of DSM-5-TR, 213
  use of terms in DSM-5-TR diagnostic process, 93–94, 278–279

Language disorder, 96–97

Latency of response, and mental status examination, 215

Learning disorders, and disruptive behavior, 39

Legal system, recording of problems with in medical record, 191

Lethargy, and inhalant intoxication, 169

Level 1 and Level 2 Cross-Cutting Symptom Measures, 70, 72, 222–223, **224–233**

Level of Personality Functioning Scale, 244

Lies and lying
  conduct disorder and, 153
  gambling disorder and, 184

Life distractions, and academic performance, 35

Lifestyle, coding of problems with in medical record, 191

Palpitations
  other hallucinogen
      intoxication and, 166
  panic disorder and, 119
Panic attacks
  anxious or avoidant
      behavior and, 49
  physical complaints and, **52**
  shorthand description of, **76**
  as specifier, 120
Panic disorder
  anxious or avoidant
      behavior and, **48,** 49
  DSM-5-TR criteria for, 119–
      120, **200**
  DSM-5-TR severity
      measures for, **255**
Parent(s). *See also* Caregivers;
    Family
  avoidance behaviors and, 50
  behavior management
      training and, 41, **300**
  coding of relational
      problems in medical
      record, 189–190
  Early Development and
      Home Background
      form and, **237–239**
  establishment of therapeu-
      tic alliance with, 6
  Level 1 and 2 Cross-Cutting
      Symptom Measures
      and, **228–233**
  postcrisis planning for, 29–
      30
  suicidality and safety
      issues, 24–25
Paresthesia, and panic
    disorder, 120
Paroxetine, **317**
Passivity, and mental status
    examination, 216

Patient(s)
  self-care strategies for, 13
  treatment plans and goals
      of, 280–283
  use of term, viii
Patient Health Questionnaire
    (PHQ), 65, **252, 255**
Pediatric Symptom Checklist
    (PSC), 70, **251**
Perseveration, and mental
    status examination, 215
Persistent depressive
    disorder, 42, **43, 57,** 114
Persistent (chronic) motor or
    vocal tic disorder, 101
Person, use of term, viii
Personality disorders
  age at onset and diagnosis
      of, 16
  DSM-5 and categorical vs.
      dimensional models
      for diagnosis of, 243–
      245
Personality Inventory for
    DSM-5-TR, 243–245,
    246–248
Personality Trait Rating
    Form, 244
Perspiration, and stimulant
    intoxication, 178
Phencyclidine use disorder,
    164–167
Phobias, and mental status
    examination, 216. *See
    also* Fear; Social phobia;
    Specific phobia
Physiological reactions, and
    PTSD, 126
Pica, 138, **203**
Picture exchange system, 39
Play, and gender dysphoria,
    148